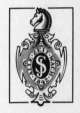

Michael Gossop

Theories
of Neurosis

With a Foreword by H. J. Eysenck

With 6 Figures

Springer-Verlag
Berlin Heidelberg New York 1981

Michael Gossop, B. A., Ph. D.
The Bethlem Royal Hospital
Drug Dependence Clinical Research
and Treatment Unit
Monks Orchard Road
Beckenham, Kent, BR3 3BX
Great Britain

ISBN 3-540-10370-8 Springer-Verlag Berlin Heidelberg New York
ISBN 0-387-10370-8 Springer-Verlag New York Heidelberg Berlin

Library of Congress Cataloging in Publication Data
Gossop, Michael, 1948 –
Theories of neurosis.
Bibliography: p.
Includes index.
1. Neuroses. I. Title. [DNLM: 1. Neuroses. 2. Psychological theory. QM 170 G68 lt]
RC 530. G58 616.85'2 80–25210

The use of registered names, trademarks, etc. in this publication does not imply, even in the
absence of a specific statement, that such names are exempt from the relevant protective laws
and regulations and therefore free for general use.
Typesetting and bookbinding: G. Appl, Wemding. Printing: aprinta, Wemding.
2125/3140-543210

The absolutely central problem in neurosis . . . is a paradox – the paradox of behaviour which is at one and the same time self-perpetuating and self-defeating.
O. H. Mowrer

The knowledge which we have that is objective and compelling has only limited extent and beyond this the individual's comprehension and attitude towards himself make endless progression.
Karl Jaspers
(translated by J. Hoenig and M. W. Hamilton)

Foreword

In view of the practical importance of neurotic disorders (with something like one-third of the population suffering such disturbances at some time of their lives) and the equally great theoretical importance of types of behaviour that clearly seem to contradict both common sense and the law of effect, one might have expected that psychologists would develop consistent and testable theories of neurosis and that there would be many textbooks outlining these theories and describing the experiments done to test them. Oddly enough nothing of the kind seems to have happened. There is a dearth of theories of neurosis; those that do exist are not usually put in a readily testable form, and the amount of research that has been done in order to test these theories is nothing like as large as one might have hoped. Nor are there many books setting out the various theories, the arguments for and against and the empirical evidence; in fact, this may be the only book to have undertaken this task in the past 20 or 30 years.

It is fortunate that the author has succeeded in what is an extremely difficult and complex task. He has examined issues and theories dispassionately and impartially, has clarified the contradictions inherent in most theories and has wisely refused to come to any kind of final judgment about the adequacy of the given theories. His aim has been to give a scholarly presentation of the most widely held theories and the evidence favouring or faulting them; in this attempt he has admirably succeeded. Only those who have tried to teach courses in this field will know the difficulties that he must have encountered and will be able to admire the ingenuity with which he has surmounted them.

The book will thus be a godsend for academics who have to teach courses in clinical or abnormal psychology, but it will also be welcomed by psychiatrists, clinical practitioners in psychology and indeed all whose business is with neurotic patients. Unless they are so taken up with one particular theory that they cannot believe that other theories too might contribute something useful, they will find here a clear statement of alternatives and a critical discussion of both the advantages and disadvantages of different theories. The book thus makes an important and indeed unique contribution to a topic that has been probably even more confused than most in the general field of psychology. The author cannot give us the right answer, but at least he will help us to ask the right questions. That is an important contribution, and the book will undoubtedly become a classic, to be revised and reprinted many times as our knowledge advances. One's only regret can be that it was not written many years ago!

November 1980   H. J. Eysenck

Contents

X   Contents

Contents   XI

Acknowledgements

In preparing this book I was helped in different ways by many of my friends and colleagues. I am particularly indebted to Hans Eysenck, who pointed out the need for a book of this sort and who provided constant help and encouragement during the time that I was struggling to write the book. I would also like to thank Dr. J. Birley, Professor Dick Eiser, Dr. Michael Feldman, Professor Walter Mischel, Professor O. H. Mowrer and Dr. Gudrun Sartory for their comments upon drafts of various chapters and for drawing my attention to work of which I would otherwise have remained unaware. Finally, I am grateful to Janet Chesson and Nan Allen for being so patient with me and for typing out the manuscript so meticulously.

Introduction

Among the most common psychological disorders are those that have traditionally been included within the category of 'neurosis'. There are a number of difficulties (both practical and theoretical) which prevent us from making any precise estimate of how many people are affected by one or other of the neurotic disorders; but even the most conservative estimates suggest that several million people must be incapacitated by them. Some of the less restrained estimates have suggested that as many as 50% of the population may at some time be affected. Whichever figure one chooses to accept, it is clear that neurotic behaviour cannot be regarded as something that is isolated from everyday life, or that is unusual. Large numbers of people are seriously affected by the neurotic disorders, and few of us are entirely free from some minor 'neurotic' reaction. Theories of neurosis play an important part in our understanding of human activity and should not be seen as relevant only to the behaviour of a small number of disturbed individuals.

The manifestations of the neurotic disorders have, of course, been obvious for centuries, though it is only comparatively recently that they have been formulated in the way in which we now recognise them, and the theories that are presented in this book are all of comparatively recent origin. The most venerable, and in a general sense, probably the most influential theory of neurosis still in current use is Freudian psycho-analysis. Freud's extensive contributions are dated from 1886 to his death in 1939, but his influence still dominates psychiatric approaches to neurosis. It is an interesting footnote to the study of neurosis that the concept of anxiety, which plays such a central role in most formulations of the neuroses, is itself attributable to Freud's writings. In 1894 Freud described anxiety neurosis as a syndrome distinct from neurasthenia, though the concept did not achieve the popularity that it currently enjoys amongst psychologists until much later. Again it was one of Freud's books, 'The Problem of Anxiety' (1936), that was largely responsible for extending its usage.

Insofar as the various neurotic disorders have a common feature, this is usually thought to be their involvement with anxiety; and in this respect some theories of neurosis are largely theories of anxiety. In some disorders, anxiety is the central and dominant feature – as in anxiety neurosis itself, where the anxiety appears as a generalised feeling of dread which contaminates almost all aspects of the person's life. In other cases, the anxiety is not free floating in this way, but is much more closely linked to specific objects or events, as in certain phobic disorders. Several theories have also regarded the behaviour rituals and compulsive thoughts that characterise the obsessional and compulsive states as being a sort of defence against the painful experience of anxiety. Such other neuroses as the conversion and dissociative disorders might appear to be less closely involved with anxiety, though anxiety is again involved as a central factor in the explanations offered by a number of different theories. Of the traditional neurotic disorders, the one that seems to be least directly related to anxiety is neurotic or reactive depression.

The neuroses are of immense clinical and theoretical importance to psychology and medicine. Because of this, it is unusual that there is no single source to which the student can turn for a survey of the different theories. Any reader who wishes to familiarise himself with a wider perspective upon the neuroses than that provided by a single theory must refer to the original material. And whereas there is no substitute for reading the original works of particular authors, over such a vast field as that covered by the neuroses, the enormity of the task must have deterred a great many readers from all but the most cursory inspection of alternative accounts to their own. By presenting an outline of each of the different theories of neurosis within a single volume, it is hoped that this book will provide the reader with a better understanding both of the neurotic disorders themselves and of the relative strength and weakness of the different theories.

The material presented in the book is necessarily selective, and the problem of selection proved to be a general difficulty throughout the preparation of the book. It was often difficult to decide what to include and what to leave out. This was a particular problem in the case of the empirical work relating to the neuroses that has appeared in the journals. There seemed to be limitless amounts of this sort of material, though its relevance to a book of this sort was, in many cases, very difficult to assess. There were also problems of selection in relationship to the theories. Some, like psycho-analysis and the conditioning models of neurosis, demanded inclusion. Others made less compelling demands for inclusion. The post-Freudian psycho-analytic theories could have been given more attention than they have in this book. The views of Melanie Klein, for instance, which have been so influential amongst British analysts, receive virtually no consideration. On the whole, it was felt that a discussion of the Freudian system itself (particularly when presented in conjunction with the views of Horney, Fromm and Adler) was adequate to give the reader an idea of the sort of explanation that psycho-analysts use in this context. I hope that any omissions will be offset by the advantages of presenting the different theories within a single volume.

The book deals with material which should be useful both to undergraduates with a special interest in abnormal psychology and to post-graduate and qualified psychologists and psychiatrists. Indeed, it is to be hoped that many others who are professionally involved with individuals suffering from neurotic difficulties will find the book useful (though a certain minimum familiarity with the concepts of psychology is assumed).

The book is divided into two parts. Part I provides the framework within which the theories are set. The first chapter provides an historical introduction to the concept of neurosis itself and describes the emergence of the different formulations of the neurotic disorders over the past two centuries. Chapters 2 and 3 extend this discussion. Chapter 2 deals with the way in which the specific neurotic disorders are currently formulated. Discussions of this sort have usually been based upon the nosological systems of psychiatry, and these are taken as the starting point for the present analysis. Chapter 2 also deals more widely with the problems inherent in different systems of classification and the difficulties of diagnosis. The final chapter of Part I examines the relationship of the concept of neurosis to two other general concepts which underpin any approach to abnormal psychology – those of normality and psychosis.

The second (and major) part of the book presents the theories themselves. These come in all shapes and sizes. In some cases they are recognisable as theories; in other cases they are more like a collection of studies linked together by a particular view of human behaviour. Nonetheless, in their own way each provides a particular perspective upon the sort of problem that is being presented, a particular formulation of the neurotic disorder itself and a particular sort of explanation of that disorder.

The traditional approach to psychological disorders over the past 200 years or so has been based upon medical assumptions. This medical (or disease) model leads us to think in terms of mental illness, of the aetiology and course of illnesses and of 'patients' and 'therapists'; and whatever defects there are in such concepts, it is still difficult to avoid their pervasive influence. Psycho-dynamic theories of neurosis represent one expression (albeit an unusual one) of the medical model. In this case the pathology of intrapsychic rather than physical, but nonetheless disordered unconscious psychological processes is thought to cause the neuroses, in the same sort of way that the medical model traces physical symptoms to an underlying physical disorder.

Personality theories have always had an appeal of their own in abnormal psychology. Trait theory represents a different attempt to explain the neuroses in personality terms, though the idea of a trait, like so many concepts in psychology, is somewhat elusive. Trait theorists have sought to identify the patterns of behaviour that remain relatively consistent for each individual over a period of time and in different situations. It has been suggested that trait theories are, therefore, descriptive rather than causal, though the conclusions of trait theorists have been translated into causal explanations of behaviour. In recent years there has been a revival of criticism directed against the most basic assumptions of trait theory, namely those concerning the cross-situational consistency of behaviour.

The work of several trait theorists has been closely linked to further assumptions about the physiological basis of personality. Attempts to explain neurotic disorders in physiological and genetic terms are as old as the concept of neurosis itself. Ever since Cullen's formulation, different psychologists and physicians have investigated these aspects of the disorders, and the search for biological causes of neurosis could be seen as another reflection of the medical tradition.

A quite different tradition, but one with an even longer history, has sought to explain behaviour by relating it to external, environmental factors. This position was first stated as far back as 3000 years ago by Homer. The impact of such views upon current psychologists, however, owes more to the work of Pavlov, Watson, Thorndike and Skinner in the early part of this century. The conditioning accounts of neurosis are still vigorous, and the work of the behaviour therapists has had a profound impact upon psychological medicine. But like each of the attempts to explain the neuroses, the conditioning theories face their own theoretical and conceptual problems. It is interesting to note that among their most vocal critics have been other learning theorists who favour a more molar, social and cognitive approach. Finally there are those sociological critics who have argued that psychology and psychiatry have too often failed to take into account those social forces which operate independently of the individual. Societal reactance (labelling) theory is one of the better-known attempts to explain the development and maintenance of psychological disorders in such terms.

Each of these theories of neurosis carries with it certain implications for treatment. The same set of behavioural symptoms look entirely different when seen as a maladaptive learned response, as an expression of unconscious intrapsychic conflicts or as a function of social expectations; and the ways in which the clinician might try to help the person who presents with such symptoms will depend upon his theoretical inclinations. The neuroses are inaccessible except through some set of theoretical assumptions (albeit implicit and unstated). For this reason, if for no other, it is important for the clinician to maintain an interest in the theoretical, as well as the more obviously 'clinical', aspects of his work. Some of the theories are closely related to specific treatment procedures or approaches. Psycho-analysis, for instance, functions simultaneously as a theory of neurosis and as a method of treatment. It is, however, beyond the scope of this book to discuss in any detail the techniques of treatment that have been applied to the neurotic disorders. It is even further beyond the scope of the book to attempt to evaluate the effectiveness of such treatments. But since it proved impossible to avoid any discussion of treatment issues, several chapters do contain a brief discussion of some of the clinical implications of a particular theory.

Psychologists generally show a regrettable lack of interest in the history of their discipline. Sometimes this is based upon a naive view of research as a sort of cumulative process which progressively increases our understanding of psychological problems. Unfortunately, what were thought to be advances quite often turn out to be evasions; and problems that were thought to have been solved re-emerge years later to puzzle other generations of psychologists. The advantage of a wider, historical perspective is that it can help to draw attention to the biases and omissions of current research, as well as illuminating the reasons why certain other issues should have achieved a more central status. As psychology becomes more and more specialised (which is itself an historical rather than a logical development), it becomes increasingly difficult to maintain any overall perspective upon certain problems in the face of this diversity. Specialised research frequently produces more specialised research, and the larger issues which stimulated the research in the first place become obscured. In an area such as that covered by the term 'neurosis', so many different disciplines have made their own distinctive contributions that an historical perspective is especially useful to counteract the dangers of treating one approach to the problem as if it were the only legitimate approach. There are historical as well as scientific reasons for the concepts and theories of psychology.

Part I

The Concept of Neurosis

1. Historical Background

Abnormal forms of human behaviour have existed for as long as records have been kept, though the history of abnormal psychology is not necessarily related to that of medicine. Mora (1967) has suggested that the earliest concepts of mental disorders were probably influenced by universal beliefs in supernatural phenomena, and specifically by a belief in ancestral spirits. For this reason the first models of abnormal behaviour were generally of a religious nature, the mentally disturbed person being seen as powerful and supernormal. In such models it was usually assumed that medicine had no power over the 'possessed' individual, and even that it had no right to deal with such people (Zilboorg and Henry 1941).

In the Neolithic Age, between about 10000 and 7000 B. C., certain diseases (for instance convulsive disorders) appear to have been treated by trepanation of the skull (Kaplan and Kaplan 1956). This operation was probably performed in order to allow the evil spirit to escape through the hole in the head. Also, there are accounts in the Bible (I Samuel) of King Saul's possession by evil spirits, and Herodotus describes how an insane king was confined and eventually committed suicide. Hippocrates (born around the year 460 B. C.) viewed mental disorders from a physical standpoint and saw the brain as the seat of such disorders. He proposed that the four elements and the four bodily humours could provide a basis for the understanding of such phenomena. Diseases were seen in terms of imbalance in the elements and humours, and this view of pathology lived on until the seventeenth century; indeed in a much modified form its influence is still with us (see for instance Pavlov 1955; Eysenck 1957).

Among the achievements credited to Hippocrates are his emphasis on natural causes, his astute clinical observations, his attempts at classifications and diagnosis, his focus on the role of the brain, and his psychological view. All these achievements are consistent with contemporary viewpoints (Ullman and Krasner 1969).

However, with the possible exception of Galen, who lived between around 130 A. D. and 200 A. D., there were few developments until comparatively recently that add to our understanding of mental disorders. Christian theology developed a view of mental life which divorced it from any significant dependence upon the body, and mental disturbances were again seen as manifestations of supernatural agencies – generally possession by demons. Those who were identified as insane within such a system were often treated worse than criminals. From the point of view of the abnormal psychologist, one of the distinguishing features of the Middle Ages is the dominant role which the clergy held in the designation and treatment of mental disorders; and in particular the events that have received most attention are the witch-hunts. These have been singled out as significant historical events in the evolution of psychiatry, though for very different reasons, by such writers as Szasz (1961), Schoeneman (1977) and Zilboorg and Henry (1941).

1.1 Neurosis

Thomas Sydenham (1624–1689) drew particular attention to the importance of differentiating between diseases and pioneered the idea of a specific pathology underlying each disease. He was also one of the first physicians to draw attention to the symptoms of neurosis. Although not specifically interested in disorders of the mind, he described in detail some of the neurotic and hysterical symptoms and noted the frequency with which they appeared in his patients. Until this time, those interested in abnormal psychology had tended to focus almost exclusively upon the more dramatic cases of psychosis.

The term 'neurosis' appears to have been first used by William Cullen in his *Nosology,* which was published in 1769. In this work, he classified all diseases according to their symptoms. The class 'neuroses' was used to refer to what we might to-day call neurological, psychosomatic, neurotic and psychotic disorders (Knoff 1970). They were diseases for which there was no known localised pathology or fever, and they included such diverse conditions as apoplexy, palsy, hypochondriasis, epilepsy, palpitation, asthma, hysteria and hydrophobia (Cullen 1781).

According to Cullen, the concepts of nervous energy and of irritability of the nervous system were of particular importance. In the course of time, many of Cullen's neuroses were reclassified as neurological and systemic diseases, but the term retained much of the notion of disordered nerve function without structural pathology for the next century. The modern usage which denotes minor psychological disorders is in many ways diametrically opposed to Cullen's use of the term (Hunter and Macalpine 1970).

From Cullen, the official psychiatry of neuroses was mostly practised by neurologists, and the term 'neurosis' referred to any somatic disorder of the nerves or of nerve function. Such disorders would now be thought of in terms of neuropathy. Almost the last commitment to the concept of neurosis as nervous disease was made by G. M. Beard, who first described neurasthenia as a clinical entity (though the term was first introduced by either Van Dusen or Maynes). Macmillan (1976) has pointed out how Freud derived his own concept of neurasthenia from that of Beard, who regarded it as a disorder characterised by general malaise, poor appetite, back pain, neuralgic pains, hypochondriasis, persistent headaches and similar complaints which occur in the absence of anaemia or organic illness (Beard 1869). Beard suggested that the primary cause of this condition was a distrubance of the balance between nerve waste and repair, which leads to an unstable and weakened nerve force. In his original statements, Beard appears to have believed that phosphorus deficiency was the major cause, though such suggestions are omitted from his later theories.

At about the same time, Mesmer was extending the tradition of the 'magnetisers' in his studies of hypnotism, and John Elliotson, a physician at St. Thomas' Hospital, London, was later to advocate the use of hypnotism in the treatment of hysteria (hysterical paralysis). Another important historical development came with Charcot's interest in this phenomenon of hysteria. During the latter part of the nineteenth century, hysterical disorders became a prominent phenomenon in psychiatry (though they showed a rapid and mysterious decline after 1900). Hysteria had been considered a strange and incomprehensible disease for centuries. Early conceptions regarded it as a physical illness confined to females, with its origin in the uterus; and a belief in the sexual psychogenesis of hysteria still persists in various forms.

In the early 1850s, Briquet made one of the first systematic studies of hysteria, which he came to regard as a neurosis of the brain with a strong hereditary component. Charcot based his concept of hysteria on that of Briquet and extended his investigations of the disorder. One of Charcot's great achievements was his investigation of traumatic paralyses, and in his studies between 1884–5 he showed the similarity between these conditions and the hysterical paralyses and reproduced similar effects under hypnosis. In 1892 he distinguished 'hysterical amnesia' from 'organic amnesia' and earned from the public the curious title of Napoleon of the Neuroses (Ellenberger 1970).

Among Charcot's failings were his over-enthusiastic extension of neurological methods into this field and his excessive concern with the specification of disease entities. Both of these features were criticised by Janet (1895). Charcot was also one of the first to label the hysterical patient as 'sick' in the medical sense of the term, a development which some writers (e. g. Szasz 1961) consider to be as detrimental as it was significant, since from this it followed that the status of such people was profoundly altered. Prior to this reconceptualisation, any physician who considered an hysteric to be sick was being fooled, whereas now the doctor could be commended for his diagnostic acumen in spotting such hysterics.

One result of the work of Charcot (together with that of Bernheim) was the release of a new impetus in psychiatry, and the neuroses were increasingly included within the respectable domain of medicine. Among those who were profoundly influenced by their work were Pierre Janet and Sigmund Freud.

Janet began his research with hysterical patients, but widened his interests to include other neuroses. He attempted to bring a greater coherence to these disorders and prepared a theory of neuroses, grouping them according to their dynamics. These ideas are summarised in his *Neuroses* (1909). He distinguished between two basic neurotic conditions – hysteria and psychasthenia, preferring the term 'psychasthenia' to 'neurasthenia' in order to avoid the implications of neurological dysfunction.

His concept of hysteria was divided into two parts and differentiated the accidental or contingent symptoms from the stigmata or basic symptoms. The accidental symptoms were thought to depend upon subconscious fixed ideas, and the stigmata were due to what Janet termed a narrowing of the field of consciousness. He rejected the purely neurological theory as well as the theory that hysterical symptoms were faked, and, following Charcot, regarded hysteria as a psychogenic disease.

Psychasthenia was also thought to include two levels of symptoms. The superficial symptoms included psychasthenic crises, acute anxiety states and obsessional and phobic disorders; and at the 'deeper' level, Janet described a basic disturbance in the individual's relationship with reality. In both the hysterical and the psychasthenic neuroses, Janet regarded the neurotic disposition as an important factor and described the inherited constitutional weaknesses of the nervous system in neurotic patients. It was, however, his dynamic theory that had the most significant influence upon current thought, mainly through its impact upon psycho-analysis. Both Jung and Adler acknowledged Janet's influence upon their work, and although Freud in his later work came to emphasise the differences between his own system and that of Janet, there is good reason to believe that Freud too owed a good deal to Janet's influence. This question of Janet's influence upon psycho-analysis is discussed later in this chapter (see The Psycho-dynamic Model).

Jaspers' *Allgemeine Psychopathologie* (General Psychopathology) first appeared in 1913 and has had a profound effect upon thinking in abnormal psychology, though it was not translated into English until half a century later (by Hoenig and Hamilton in 1963). One of Jaspers' explicit aims was to produce a systematized approach in terms of methods in psychopathology and to build a common terminology. He distinguishes three groups of disorders. Group I includes such diseases as cerebral trauma, cerebral tumours, acute infections (meningitis for instance) and GPI (General paralysis of the insane) for which there are known somatic events; in Group II we find the three major psychoses and in Group III what he refers to as Psychopathien, the personality disorders (including the neuroses, such as anxiety states, phobias, hysterical disorders, obsessive-compulsive disorders and reactive depression. Indeed, Jaspers' concept of the neuroses includes all the conditions included within the contemporary psychiatric systems of classification, though he tends to make certain distinctions which are not currently seen – such as that between psychasthenia and neurasthenia).

The first group of diseases satisfies the usual requirement of real disease entities, but it is the mental and affective disorders represented by the psychoses and the personality disorders which present the main problem in abnormal psychology. Jaspers suggests that one must . . . assume that many of these psychoses have a somatic base which one day will be known (*General Psychopathology* 1972). Having made this point, Jaspers goes on to propose the possible division of psychopathological events into two classes, Groups I and III. Those that may be classified as organic disorders with somatic origins would comprise one group, and those that are disorders of living would comprise the other. The psychoses may be considered to be of rather uncertain status – hovering somewhere between Groups I and III, in the absence of adequate or complete knowledge of their origins. When they are better understood they might be expected to fall into either one or the other of the two main categories. More recently, a similar proposal has been made by Hans Eysenck (1975).

For the present purposes, it is Jaspers' ideas about the neuroses that are the most interesting. Of the Group III disorders he says that classification poses very difficult problems. Diagnostic efforts have got lost in the establishment of individual facts, mechanisms, states and characteristics. However, he points out how important it is to distinguish between psychological *reactions* and *types of personality*.

To illustrate the significance of this point, Jaspers refers to the work of Schultz, who attempted to distinguish between the generally neurotic personality and the individual neuroses. In some cases the neurotic symptoms may occur in relative isolation. In the neurotic individual, on the other hand, it is sometimes found that a large number of different neurotic features occur and that these differ both in quantity and quality and may be constantly changing. Schultz gives the name *exogenous* neuroses to the phenomena which are conditioned by external stimuli and which are capable of being cured by environmental means. To the 'deeper' disorders which are a result of well-established personality features he gives the name *nuclear* or *core neuroses*. These nuclear or core neuroses are regarded as extremely difficult for the therapist to deal with, being curable only very slowly through personality development. For this latter type of disorder, Schultz suggests that Freudian or Jungian therapies may be appropriate. Unfortunately, as Jasper points out, these diagnostic categories were too reliant upon subsequent therapeutic outcome. If the neuroses responded to environmental manipulation they were exogenous; if they did not, and more lengthy psychotherapeutic procedures were needed, then this indicated the presence of nuclear neuroses based upon personality disturbance. It is this circularity which contains the essential weakness of such a diagnostic scheme, and Jaspers suggests that in an area that is so vague, post hoc procedures of this kind are of very limited value in terms of concrete results. "In the last resort probably all neuroses point to a nuclear neurosis and even the severest neurosis will still allow simple exogenous neuroses to arise" *(General Psychopathology)*.

Jaspers argues that for the disorders of Group III no proper diagnosis can be made, though it is possible to separate the disorders into a large enough number of descriptive type-groupings. Apart from this, the best that can be achieved is an extensive analysis of the case which deals with each of the specific personality, social and phenomenological features. Since Cullen first coined the term 'neurosis', its meaning has been continually changing. Marks (1973[a]) describes two different meanings. In its first connotation, it has been used to describe syndromes like anxiety states, depression, phobic disorders, obsessional states and hysterical symptoms. But in its wider meaning, the term has been used to describe persistent maladaptive behaviour, especially in an interpersonal context, which is distressing to the person concerned.

The varying and imprecise definitions that have been offered have led to some serious problems in psychological medicine. They have prevented direct comparisons of the results of different research studies and caused disagreement between clinicians that have been at least partly due to semantic confusion. Culpin (1962) expressed his exasperation with the term, which he describes as" . . . that final triumph of the nineteenth century . . . an embodiment of pseudo-physiology, unsound metaphysics, and moral condemnation". But apart from developments in the concept of neurosis itself, other profound changes were taking place in abnormal psychology during this period. These were also to have important effects upon professional attitudes and approaches to be neurotic disorders.

1.2 The Organic Model

The earliest statements of this position were made by Hippocrates, the father of medicine, who argued that certain mental disorders were diseases of the brain. A little later, Lucretius in *De Rerum Natura* pursued the same theme, that mental disorders were different from normal, healthy behaviour and were to be regarded in the same way as physical diseases. From a contemporary viewpoint, the organic model (sometimes also referred to as the medical model, though the two are not strictly synonymous) is usually traced back to the eighteenth century. Since then it has occupied a dominant position in psychiatry and has had a massive influence upon the development of research and clinical practice in psychological medicine.

Wilhelm Griesinger's book, *Pathology and Therapy of Mental Diseases,* was published in 1845 and soon became accepted as the most authoritative work in its field. Griesinger maintained that mental disorders could only be explained in terms of physical changes which occurred in the nervous system, and he considered the brain and its pathology to be the essential feature of all mental illnesses. For this reason he argued that it was futile for the psychiatrist to pay too much attention to the problems of psychological description and classification, since such phenomena were of only secondary importance as correlates of the illness.

Henry Maudsley (1835–1918), one of the most influential British psychiatrists of his day, was also committed to the notion of insanity as a bodily disease. He differs from earlier writers in his emphasis upon chemical determinants of psychological phenomena. Lewis (1951) quotes Maudsley's views on this.

How different the world looks according as the liver is or is not acting well. Doubt, despair, even suicide on the one hand; faith, hope, and life-love on the other hand; these are determined respectively by some minute and subtile organic compound which has been either insufficiently or sufficiently manipulated before its discharge into the bloodstream.

Maudsley appears also to have accepted that these 'diseases' were incurable, refusing for instance to classify those patients who were well on discharge from hospital as 'recovered'.

At this time, the concept of neurosis was still at a comparatively early stage of development. Maudsley wrote of three neuroses – the epileptic, the insane and the criminal neuroses – and saw these in terms of inherited predispositions. 'The sufferer from any one of these neuroses represents an initial form of degeneracy . . . and life to him will be a hard struggle against the radical bias of his nature' (Maudsley 1899). This predisposition he referred to as the insane temperament *(Neurosis spasmodica* or *Neurosis insana),* that is, a lack of balance between the different nerve centres and their tendency to instability and to disruptive action. The neurotic person could not be said to be mad, but manifested a lesser degree of disturbance and was seen in terms of eccentricity or strangeness, and this suggestion that neurosis represents a less extreme disturbance than the psychotic disorders, and that one of the distinguishing features of the neuroses is that the individual retains some contact with reality, has been an enduring theme of the various concepts of neurosis. These issues are discussed at greater length later in the book. Maudsley also suggested that the distinctions between the neuroses were vague and ill-defined, and that the different nervous diseases were very closely related.

Another figure whose work has had a profound influence on the history of psychiatry is Emil Kraeplin (1856–1926). The publication of his *Psychiatrie* and its subsequent translation into English provided a foundation for the current nosological systems of psychiatry, and Slater and Roth (1974) have suggested that modern psychiatry begins with Kraeplin. In his general approach, Kraeplin attempted to show that mental illnesses are like physical illnesses, in that they run a typical and predictable course from their onset to their conclusion. He placed great value on prognosis – the final outcome of the illness. Unfortunately, this emphasis on prognosis carried with it the idea that certain mental disorders had an unfavourable prognosis, as in the case of dementia praecox, which Kraeplin regarded as an incurable condition. In this way, Kraeplin's views sometimes led to a rather pessimistic and predetermined view of certain disorders.

In this objective – to establish a conception of mental disorders as diseases in exactly the same sense that disorders such as tuberculosis and pneumonia were diseases – Kraeplin was successful. A contemporary of Kraeplin argued that any classification which is based upon clinical symptomatology is necessarily unsatisfactory, because the indications of one form of disease frequently coincide with those of another. Equally, an aetiological basis is unsatisfactory, since the fundamental causation is frequently unknown, and the best approach is a classification dependent upon 'the *morbid anatomy,* for when the pathology of a disease has once been recognised, the course can be predicted with some certainty, and the treatment instituted rests upon a solid foundation' (Berkley 1901).

Kraeplin also succeeded in having mental diseases accepted as an appropriate area for the intervention of medical science (Thomson 1968). Indeed psychiatry became more completely integrated with medicine at this particular period than at any previous time.

In the editor's preface to the 1906 translation of Kraeplin's *Lectures on Clinical Psychiatry,* Johnstone voiced his optimism about recent developments in which a possible physical basis for certain mental disorders had been proposed. Johnstone was referring specifically to the work associating general paralysis of the insane with a bacillus. In 1897 a crucial experiment had been conducted by Richard von Krafft-Ebing, a Viennese psychiatrist, which demonstrated the relationship between syphilis and paresis. The Wasserman test was devised in 1906; and rather later, in 1913, the presence of the spirochete causing syphilis was discovered in the brain of paretic patients during post-mortem examinations by Noguchi and Moore. This discovery of the cause of general paresis had a considerable effect on the study of abnormal behaviour, in that it gave massive support to the organic model. Since the physical basis of syphilis had been discovered, many psychiatrists were reinforced in their belief that such a basis would eventually be found for all forms of abnormal behaviour.

But whereas this event gave impetus to the organic model, the work of Griesinger and Kraeplin played a large part in establishing the tradition. Zilboorg and Henry (1941) have commented:

> It was medicine which rose to conquer the field of psychiatry. But, curiously enough, medicine was quite unwilling to accept, was even harshly opposed to, psychotherapy; it was the sphere of diseases which it was anxious to capture, but it seemed unable to abandon the tradition of the dissecting room, the apothecary, or the kitchen and insisted upon anatomy, drugs, and diet. Medicine captured psychiatry, brought it into its scientific empire, and offered it rights of citizenship only on the condition that it learn the language and submit to the administration. Medicine refused to have psychology admitted; any appearance of psychology was considered an intrusion or an illegal importation (pp 354–355).

By the end of the nineteenth century and largely through Kraeplin's influence, much of the confusion surrounding psychological disturbances had apparently been resolved. The categorisation which clearly delineated different disease entities had been established, and this system of classification remains the most potent influence upon present-day psychiatric nosology.

Kraeplin's position is that of traditional medical practice; he saw psychiatric conditions as diseases in the full sense of the term, each with a specific aetiology, pathology, symptomatology and course of its own. Kraeplin insisted, for instance, upon definite clinical diagnoses. Diagnosis was deemed to be vital, since it gave the correct basis for the prognosis of the illness. In his text *Psychiatrie* he comments:

> What has convinced me more than anything else of the superiority of the clinical methods here used over the traditional diagnostic methods is the certainty with which we are able, on the basis of our concept of disease, to predict the future course of events, and the ease with which the student can orient himself under this guidance in the difficult field of psychiatry (Kraeplin 1896).[1]

But his search for structural lesions in the brain or for biochemical dysfunction yielded no satisfactory gains in understanding. Kraeplin's own inference in the face of his failure to determine organic factors at the root of his illnesses was that their aetiology and pathology depended upon hereditary and constitutional factors of an unknown kind. However, Kraeplin's influence may be said to have had its greatest effect in terms of his concept of

---

1 "Was mir aber die Überlegenheit des hier befolgten klinischen Verfahrens über die herkömmliche Diagnostik unzweifelhaft dargetan hat, das ist die Sicherheit, mit welcher wir auf Grund unserer Krankheitsbegriffe den zukünftigen Gang der Dinge vorauszusagen im Stande sind."

psychosis. He succeeded in establishing two new categories of 'functional psychoses' – manic depressive illness and dementia praecox. The neurotic disorders, on the other hand, received rather less attention. In his *Lectures on Clinical Psychiatry* (1906), for instance, the only type of neurotic disorder that is discussed is hysteria. This failure to differentiate the neuroses from the psychotic disorders represents one of the great deficiencies of Kraeplin's work.

The various theories of psychopathology that have been proposed since Griesinger have implicated almost all biological systems in the causation of mental illness. There are, however, certain repetitive themes. Sheflen (1958) notes the tenacity of the conviction that some lesion or somatic dysfunction causes mental illness, despite the general paucity of empirical support for any such belief. One consequence of this belief is that the pathology is frequently seen as a *passive response* to toxic metabolites, pathogens or inherited effects: also brain dysfunction and mental symptoms are seen not as correlates, but as related through cause and effect. Hunter (1973) has stated that an abnormal mental state is equivalent to a physical sign of something going wrong in the brain and that ultimately mental disorders will be shown to be caused by physical dysfunction. Like Griesinger, Hunter also directs attention away from the psychological features of the disorder, on the grounds that these psychological aspects do not constitute the disorder itself, nor even its essence or determinant, but an epiphenomenon.

In recent years there has been some dispute about this organic approach to abnormal psychology, and it has received a good deal of criticism (see for instance, Szasz 1961; Eysenck 1961). But despite the fact that several psychiatrists have denied that the model is still used, this view retains its enthusiastic advocates, and the majority of psychiatrists probably implicitly accept the model. Lazare points out how few psychiatrists explicitly identify the conceptual models that they use in their formulation of cases, and suggests that one of the important models used is in fact the medical model. This regards psychiatric illnesses as diseases like any others. For each disease, it is assumed that eventually a specific cause related to the functional anatomy of brain will be found. The physician using the medical model concerns himself with the problems of aetiology, signs and symptoms, differential diagnosis, treatment and prognosis. Knowledge of the particular syndrome or disease is assumed to determine the treatment, and although the doctor addresses his patients with proper medical respect, he keeps his distance so as to maintain his objectivity (Lazare 1973).

Dietz (1977) accepts this definition of the medical model but suggests that it is no longer the prevalent ideology among psychiatrists and has not been so probably since the 1960s. Despite this, there is still a considerable amount of support being offered. It is claimed, for instance, that the primary identity of the psychiatrist is that of a physician, and that the medical model is the most useful and appropriate for the practice of psychiatry (Foulds 1955; Ludwig 1975; Engel 1972; Ludwig and Othner 1977; Sandifer 1977).

However, there is no necessary connection between the medical model and the organic model, though the two usually go together. One psychiatrist who has stressed that the two are different is Clare (1976), who asserts that the medical model is more broadly based than the organic model, and that it takes into account both environmental and individual factors. Nonetheless, Clare accepts the notion of underlying causes, which is common to both. It is this feature of the two models that has most significance to this discussion of abnormal psychology.

Although the underlying cause is usually inferred to be some sort of physical disease entity, in some special cases the medical model is applied in an allegorical sense. The most important example of this concerns Freudian systems of psycho-analysis. Psycho-analysis, like the literal, organic version of the medical model, relies upon this notion of *underlying causes*. The abnormal behaviour itself is seen as the symptomatic expression of the 'deeper' pathogenic condition, and 'treatment' should be geared to the elimination of this underlying disorder. The 'superficial' behavioural problems are related to their cause in the same way that elevation of fever or white corpuscle count are manifestations of infection in the body (Stuart 1970). Craighead et al. (1976) refer to this as the *quasi-medical model* of abnormal behaviour.

1.3 The Psycho-dynamic Model and the Concept of Intrapsychic Conflict

The psycho-dynamic model of abnormal behaviour assumes the existence of hypothetical 'psychological diseases'. Although these are not usually considered to be real entities, they are assumed to function in a similar manner to the systemic or traumatic disorders of the organic model. Neurotic symptoms are seen as the symbolic expression of some sort of underlying conflict, and the symptoms themselves are assumed to have deeper psychological significance (Blum 1966; Laughlin 1967).

The psycho-dynamic model can be traced back to Ancient Greece, and Ducey and Simon (1975) have described the development of ideas about the determinants of mental life from the time of Homer to that of Plato – from roughly the eighth to the fourth centuries B. C. The Platonic position contains a number of remarkable similarities to current psycho-dynamic models of intrapsychic conflict, and Freud himself always acknowledged his debt to Plato and the Greek tragedians. Plato, for instance, was one of the first to present a unified concept of the sexual instinct, and both Plato and Freud taught the original bisexuality of the human being and the sublimation of the sexual instinct. The earlier Homeric position, on the other hand, has more in common with social learning theory interpretations of neurosis. Table 1 presents some features of the two positions.

Any analogy between the positions of Homer and Plato and modern psychologists needs to be treated with some caution, since there are also massive differences. Plato, for instance, stressed that the emotions were to be subdued by reason, which differs radically from Freud's views about the essential role of the emotions. Nonetheless, it is possible that there is some direct link between the Platonic position and Freud. Freud was certainly interested in Ancient Greece. This is reflected in his choice of terms (Oedipus complex, Thanatos, Electra complex), and Simon argues that Freud's assumptions about mind, madness and the proper treatment for intrapsychic conflicts were influenced by Plato (Simon 1972, 1973).

Because of the impact that Freud's work has had upon contemporary thought, there is a tendency to equate the intrapsychic conflict model with Freudian psycho-analysis. There are, however, other important models of this sort, and Freud's originality has been somewhat overstated in accounts of the development of such ideas. The determinants of mental illness that are suggested by the dynamic schools are based upon a concept of mental energy which is not greatly different from earlier theories of nerve fluids. Beard's concept of neurasthenia relied heavily upon the idea of energy distribution; and Mesmer also thought of health as a product of the balance or imbalance of a universal physical

Table 1. Models of man in the writings of Homer and Plato. This compares the models of psychological disorder that are contained in the writings of Homer and Plato. The same issues are dealt with at greater length by Ducey and Simon (1975), Simon and Weiner (1966), Simon (1972, 1973) and Culpin (1962)

Homeric View	Platonic View
What we consider to be inner mental states are represented in concrete observable behaviour.	Primary emphasis upon the psyche as a structure, a mental apparatus, the parts of which are in conflict, each having its own interests, needs and ways of functioning. The rational (logistikon) is in opposition to the appetitive (epithumetikon).
Mental activity is not to be seen as intrinsically private and inaccessible but as amenable to observation.	
The events of a person's life constitute his identity – though this does not imply a passive and deterministic view of human nature.	Emphasis upon 'Eros' as an important driving force in human behaviour.
Identity is closely linked to family, friends and social environment.	Concept of sanity as ideal functioning. Therapy through self-knowledge, personality growth and insight.
Mental disorders are caused by external events and forces, not by internal conflict.	Emphasis upon internal life of the individual, and use of introspection as a way of knowing.
Mental disturbances can be relieved by attempts to reintegrate the person within the social group.	Mental disturbances as a result of intrapsychic conflict. Sickness of the psyche caused by the dominance of primitive forces.
	Therapy builds upon the relationship between philosopher and student.

fluid and regarded hypnosis in terms of the circulation of this fluid in the body of the hypnotised person or between the hypnotist and subject. Many of Freud's other ideas have clear historical antecedents; Ellenberger (1970) and Marx and Hillix (1963) have identified Leibniz, Bernheim, Charcot, Schopenhauer, Darwin, Fechner, Janet, Herbart and Meyer among the many influential figures to propose ideas that Freud later included within his own system.

Leibniz was the first to offer a psychological theory of the unconscious mind and to distinguish degrees of consciousness. A century later Herbart extended these ideas and introduced a dynamic conception of the conflict of unconscious forces as they struggle to reach consciousness. Herbart thought of the threshold of consciousness in terms of the conflict of a dynamic system of perceptions and memories, in which the stronger ones force down or repress the weaker. The repressed representations then continue their efforts to emerge into consciousness and often become associated with other representations in their struggle.

These concepts of conflict and repression which play such an important role in psychodynamic systems can also be traced back to Schopenhauer and Nietzsche. Schopenhauer explained insanity as being due to The Will's opposition to repellent information and its resistance to allowing this to become conscious; and Nietzsche too described repression as an active, inhibitory force. Indeed, the philosophical works of Schopenhauer and Nietzsche contain some of the closest parallels to psycho-analysis. Thomas Mann, who read Schopenhauer before he became familiar with Freud's work, described psycho-analysis as Schopenhauer translated from metaphysics into psychology. This can be seen in the striking resemblances between The Will and Freud's later concept of the unconscious. The Will was characterised as a blind, irrational driving force which determined man's behaviour, and Schopenhauer compared consciousness with the surface of the earth, the interior of which remains unconscious and unknown to us: among the irrational forces, the most powerful was the sexual instinct. The study of hypnotism had also led to a concept of the duality of the human mind and, later, to the notion of multiple subpersonalities. In his book, *The Double Ego,* Dessoir presented a statement of the former position – that the mind functioned at two separate levels, each of which had its own distinct characteristics. Dessoir called these *upper consciousness* (Oberbewußtsein) and *under consciousness* (Unterbewußtsein). It was from this tradition that Janet derived his concept of the subconscious.

The experimental investigations of perception that Fechner and Helmholtz were conducting around 1860, and their implications in terms of thresholds of consciousness, and unconscious interference with conscious processes were also potent influences upon Freud's thinking. Helmholtz (1866) coined the term *unconscious interference* to describe the relationship between perceptions and past experiences; stimuli are perceived not merely in terms of their physical properties but also in terms of their associations. Freud frequently quoted Fechner and derived certain features of his concept of mental energy and the pleasure principle from him. Fechner's comments that the difference between waking and sleep states was less one of intensity of function, but was more like the alternate presentation of the same mental activities on different theatre stages, have also been said to have formed the basis for Freud's topology of the mind (Ellenberger 1970).

Pierre Janet was the first to use the term 'subconscious', and he was also the first to publish a report of hysterical patients being cured through bringing their subconscious fixed ideas into consciousness (Janet 1891). Marcelle, a young woman of 20, showed difficulty in carrying out movements in which any sort of conscious decision was required and also displayed amnesias. Janet classified these and other symptoms according to their depth within the personality – from the most superficial, which he equated with posthypnotic suggestions, to the most profound, such as early traumatic events. Among the events noted in treatment are the substitution of symptoms and the effects of catharsis. Janet also discusses the gradual process of removing the superficial layers of delusions in order to penetrate into the deeper, more basic disturbances. As these were worked through, the patient showed considerable improvement. One of the general points made by Janet in this case is that nothing is ever lost to the human mind, though it may be hidden deep within the subconscious.

In his earlier work (e. g. Breuer and Freud 1895), Freud acknowledged Janet's influence, but later he increasingly came to deny the similarities between their two positions. In 1896, Freud called his own system 'psycho-analysis' in order to differentiate it from Janet's 'psychological analysis', and Ellenberger (1970) suggests that Freud emphasised the differences by giving a distorted account of Janet's views, asserting, for instance, that Janet's theory of hysteria was based upon the notion of 'degeneration'. Among the concepts and ideas that Freud shared with, or derived from, Janet, are the reality principle (Janet referred to this as the 'function of reality'), the role of repression (narrowing of the field of consciousness) in the aetiology of hysterical symptoms and the emphasis upon the nature of the patient-therapist relationship. But despite the similarities in their positions and the fact that Janet had made the earlier statement of some of the important features of the new psycho-dynamic theory, the slow development of interest in his own work in its academic framework contrasts with the remarkable popularity which Freud's psycho-analysis acquired. Of the period between 1905–1910, Brill (1936) commented that, 'Not only were the Freudian principles applied to the patients, but psychoanalysis seemed to obsess everybody at the clinic.'

1.4 Moral Treatment

This tradition has been largely out of favour for some time. It was superceded by the medical model, and in many ways the two conceptions of psychological disorders are quite opposed. Whereas the medical model relies heavily upon the disease concept, with its implications of physical and organic disorder, and therefore upon medical modes of intervention, both Pinel and Tuke emphasised the rational aspects of the disturbed person and looked to psychological treatments. Tuke (1813) explains his preference for moral treatment, 'attaching as I do, little importance to pharmaceutic preparations'.

Over 150 years later, the same point has been restated – that too often psychiatrists obscure the psychological and moral problems through their emphasis upon the physical and physiochemical needs of their patients (Sederer 1977).

Historically, the moral treatments are often traced back to one specific event – the 'striking off of the chains' of the patients at the Bicetre Hospital in Paris which occurred in 1793; and humanistic forms of psychiatric treatment flourished during the period following the French and American Revolutions. In his classic work *'A Treatise on Insanity'* (1801), Pinel comments,

> My experience authorises me to affirm, that there is no neccessary connection between the specific character of insanity, and the nature of its exciting cause. Among the cases of periodical mania, which I have seen and recorded in my journals, I find some which originated in a violent but unfortunate passion, others in an ungovernable ambition for fame, power or glory. Many succeeded to reverses of fortune; others were produced by devotional phrenzy; and others by an enthusiastic patriotism, unchastened by the sober and steady influence of solid judgement. The violence of maniacal paroxysms appears, likewise to be independent of the nature of the exciting cause; or to depend, at least, much more upon the constitution of the individual, – upon the different degrees of his physical and moral sensibility . . .

Pinel developed a simplified classification system which included the neuroses (after Cullen), though unlike Cullen's, Pinel's concept of hysteria and the neuroses seems to be that their importance as nervous disorders (i. e. physical disorders) was of less significance than their status as moral (i. e. psychological) disorders. King (1958) has described Pinel as providing a bridge between the nosologists of the eighteenth and twentieth centuries. But Pinel's principal concern lay with his patients and their clinical description rather than with rigid systems of classification.

Another individual whose name is associated with this approach to the treatment of the mentally disturbed individual is William Tuke, the founder of The Retreat Hospital in York. The decision to open a fund for the establishment of The Retreat almost coincided with the actions of Pinel at the Bicetre in Paris, though whereas Pinel was motivated largely by his scientific studies, the founders of The Retreat were swayed primarily by humanitarian and religious motives. Samuel Tuke has stated the aims of the managers of The Retreat. They were based upon the care and alleviation of the mental disorder 'by judicious modes of management and moral treatment'. It was recognised that "Insane persons generally possess a degree of control over their wayward propensities. Their intellectual, active and moral powers are usually rather perverted than obliterated: and it happens, not unfrequently that one faculty only is affected. The disorder is sometimes still more partial, and can only be detected by erroneous views, on one particular topic" (Samuel Tuke 1813).

In his description of the early history of The Retreat, Hunt (1932) points to certain questions posed by the proponents of moral treatment. Firstly there was the question of how the patients could be helped to control their disorder, and secondly 'by what means the general comfort of the insane is promoted'.

Both Pinel and Tuke recognised that the abnormal behaviour found among the insane was dependent to some degree upon the psychological and social environments in which such people found themselves, and their view of the causes of madness emphasised psychological factors. Indeed the term 'moral' has been regarded as synonymous with 'psychological' by Sederer (1977), who points out that the German phrase for this form of treatment – *psychologische Hilfsmittel* – means 'psychological means of help'.

Moral treatment usually involved making the patient feel comfortable, arousing his interest and forming a friendly relationship with him. Having established a relationship in a friendly atmosphere, free from restraint, the patient was then encouraged to discuss his troubles. Manual work was considered beneficial, and the patients' time was filled with purposeful activities (Bockoven 1956). This form of treatment has similarities with several of the present-day psychotherapies. Proponents of dynamic psychotherapies may find in the friendly relationships that were such an important aspect of moral treatment something suggestive of 'positive transference'. Equally, the Skinnerian behaviour therapist may see the similarities between the emphasis upon responsibility and appropriate behaviour of moral treatment and modern operant programmes. In a comparison of the therapeutic orientation of Pinel, Tuke and others such as Vincenzo Chiarugi, who was working along similar lines in Italy at this time, Mora (1967) shows that each of their approaches emphasised the healthy part of the patient's behaviour and personality, and Albee (1969) refers to moral treatment as a suitable model for contemporary psychotherapy in its emphasis upon the psychological strengths and skills of the patient, rather than upon his 'sickness'. It is easy to recognise in these features certain aspects of behaviour modification (Bandura 1969); there are also aspects of moral treatment that are closely related to what we would today call occupational therapy and recreational therapy, though any attempt to draw too close a comparison is bound to be misleading. It is probably a mistake to regard moral treatment as a specific procedure. It was much more of an attempt to create a generally favourable environment for the person, in which spontaneous recovery might take place.

Although the direct influence of moral treatment upon modern psychiatry and clinical psychology has been comparatively slight, the significance of these developments lies in their expression of the humanistic tradition, with its emphasis upon the person and his human dignity. In recent years there has been an increasing expression of dissatisfaction among psychologists with mechanistic and reductionist approaches to the explanation of human behaviour (Kagan 1967; Sanford 1965; Braginsky and Braginsky 1974; Giorgi 1970). More specifically there has also been a reaction to the inadequate and damaging social environments that exist in many psychiatric hospitals. Goffman (1961) has argued that the more progressive and medical institutions may be even more damaging than purely custodial ones, and Rosenhan (1973) has given an account of the effects of such institutions upon sane and 'normal' individuals.

In short, the demonstrations that moral treatment could provide a humane and a therapeutically effective environment were largely ignored. The medical model that replaced it relied upon

> The authoritative scientific verdict that mental illness was due to incurable brain disease (which) eliminated the belief, on which moral treatment was based, that patients were capable of responding as persons to sympathetic human understanding. Since no scientific treatment for mental illness had yet been discovered, mental hospitals became mere receptacles for the incurable (Bockoven 1956).

As such, the hospitals generally fell back upon custodial care, content to look after the physical well-being of their patients and fulfilling the dual roles of control and protection.

1.5 Learning Theory and Behaviour Therapy

In contrast to the Cartesian view that man's ideas and behaviour were dependent upon innate factors, John Locke, the English empiricist philosopher, proposed that the child's mind be regarded as a *tabula rase*. Psychological phenomena were to be regarded as a product of learning and experience. Although others had expressed this sort of view before Locke (e. g. Aristotle), Locke laid greater emphasis upon acquired behaviour than those before him.

Locke's views had particular influence on Ivan Sechenov, the founder of Russian physiology, who in his *Reflexes of the Brain* (1863) presented the argument that all forms of behaviour are reflexive in origin. Reflexes were themselves acquired through a process of associative learning, and pointing to the role of repeated presentations of stimuli in the formation of all kinds of acquired associations, Sechenov undoubtedly came close to Pavlov's conception of conditioned reflexes. Pavlov read the works of Sechenov, and they left a profound, life-long impression on his ideas.

The term 'conditioning' refers to two psychological procedures – classical conditioning and instrumental conditioning. It is the first of these, classical or respondent conditioning, which is derived from Pavlov's investigations. Pavlov was a physiologist: in his early research he was concerned with the heart and the digestive organs, and in 1904 he won the Nobel prize for his work on digestion. In his investigation of the digestive organs in dogs, Pavlov noted that the sight or odour of food could provoke the secretion of digestive juices. Pavlov used this as a vehicle for the investigation of the functions of the cerebral cortex and was the first to use the procedures and concepts of conditioning, conditioned and unconditioned stimuli, reinforcement, irradiation (stimulus generalisation) and extinction and spontaneous recovery (Gormezano and Moore 1969). In his classical experiment on the conditioned reflex, Pavlov presented the sound of a bell at the same time as food powder was given to the experimental animal. After a number of simultaneous presentations the bell alone came to elicit the salivation. The essential feature of classical conditioning is that an unconditioned stimulus (UCS), which reliably produces an unconditioned response (UCR), is presented with a conditioned stimulus (CS), which has been shown not to produce the UCR. By repeated presentations of the CS and UCS (in a specified time sequence), the CS comes to produce a response similar

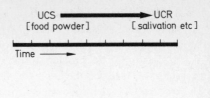

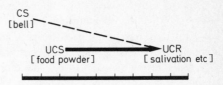

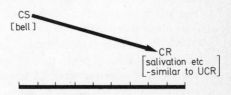

Fig. 1. The classical conditioning paradigm (Pavlovian A conditioning)

to the UCR. This is the conditioned response (CR). This procedure is sometimes referred to as *Pavlovian A conditioning* (Grant 1964) and is shown in diagrammatic presentation in Fig. 1.

In stage 1, the simple unconditioned reflex is shown. In stage 2, repeated paired presentations of the CS and UCS lead to stage 3, in which the conditioned connection is established: the CS produces the CR, which is similar but not identical to the UCR. An important feature of Pavlovian A conditioning is the *consummatory response,* in this case the ingestion of the food powder.

Of greater relevance to any consideration of the neuroses is *Pavlovian B conditioning.* In this case, events are not dependent upon the instrumental behaviour of the animal, and after conditioning the CS appears to act as a partial substitute for the UCS; that is, unlike Pavlovian A conditioning, the UCS elicits a more complete UCR. Grant (1964) suggests that this subclass of classical conditioning should be called Watsonian conditioning, after Watson and Rayner's (1920) study.

The interval between presentation of the CS and UCS is known to affect the rate of conditioning, although the exact details of the relationship between the stimuli are not fully understood. It has been suggested on the basis of the current empirical data that the optimum interval between CS and UCS is of the order of 0.5 seconds (Gormezano and Moore 1969); and it is also generally accepted that conditioning takes place most efficiently when the CS precedes the UCS. At one time Pavlov regarded backward conditioning (where the UCS precedes the CS) as an impossibility (Pavlov 1927). He later revised this opinion, but noted that under such conditions the CR was at best weak and unstable (Pavlov 1928 and Pavlov 1941).

Apart from his research into digestion and higher nervous activity in animals, Pavlov was concerned with the problems of abnormal psychology. One event which stimulated research in this field was the Leningrad flood of 1924. During the storms the animals had to be rescued from the flood waters which had penetrated the laboratory buildings, and although all the dogs were saved, they showed several unusual reactions. The conditioned responses which had been established experimentally prior to the flood disappeared; it was as if they had never been formed, and it was possible to restore them only very gradually by means of numerous repetitions. But apart from this, one of the dogs had acquired a strong aversion to the sound of the bell that had formerly been used in the laboratory as a conditioned stimulus. Pavlov seems to have regarded this form of experimental neurosis as analogous in some ways to neurasthenic disorders in humans. Frolov, who was one of Pavlov's students, writes that 'Pavlov came to the conclusion that the powerful sound, precisely because of its strength . . . reminded the dog of the flood . . . the dog had ceased to be able to bear strong stimuli, just as sick persons, neurotics, are unable to bear them' (Frolov 1938).

At about the same time, J. B. Watson in America was developing a theory of behaviour based upon this concept of the conditioned reflex. Despite its many similarities to Pavlov's work, Watson's work was done largely independently. A few years before Pavlov's observations on the reaction of his dogs to the flooding of his laboratory, J. B. Watson and Rosalie Rayner published an account of the same sort of conditioned emotional reaction as described by Pavlov in the Leningrad flood (Watson and Rayner 1920). Using an 11-month-old infant (Albert), Watson paired a neutral stimulus (a white rat) with a fear-producing stimulus (a loud noise). After only seven pairings the infant showed a completely conditioned fear response to the white rat. This conditioned response was found to generalise to similar stimuli, for instance a white rabbit, a fur coat and a Santa Claus mask. Watson and Rayner concluded that many of the phobias found in human psychopathology are true conditioned emotional responses.

Watson is usually regarded as an extreme environmentalist who felt that man's complex behaviour patterns were entirely dependent upon learning, and in one of his best-known pronouncements he asserted that, given any healthy infant, he could make the child into a doctor, a lawyer, a thief or whatever he chose through conditioning. In view of this, the comment of Watson and Rayner that 'One may possibly have to believe that such persistence of early conditioned responses will be found only in persons who are constitutionally inferior' is interesting in its suggestion that individual constitutional differences may have some effect on the development of neurotic responses. This aspect of individual differences in responsiveness, however, was particularly emphasised by Pavlov, who recognised three basic properties of nervous function – *strength, balance* and *lability*. On the basis of these, Pavlov used a typology similar to that of Hippocrates, whose influence he acknowledges (Pavlov 1955).

Around the beginning of the 1920s Pavlov came to the conclusion that the 'strength' of the nervous system plays a crucial role in the establishment of individual differences (Nebylitsyn 1964): the basis for Pavlov's typology lay in his ideas concerning the extreme reactivity and rapid exhaustability of cortical cells. As a result of repeated exposure to a conditioned stimulus, the cells of the hemispheres were thought to pass into an inhibitory state. Pavlov developed the theory that different animals exhibited different degrees of reactivity to stimulation and spoke of the ease with which excitation or inhibition built up within the nervous system as an index of its strength or weakness. The 'balance' within the nervous system depended upon the equality or inequality of the two processes of excitation and inhibition.

These properties were closely related to the sort of disorder that an animal or person might develop. In those cases where there was an imbalance between the excitatory and inhibitory processes, experimental neuroses could be produced with relative ease. The excitatory type of animal loses much of its ability for inhibition and becomes unusually excited and agitated, whereas the inhibitory type becomes excessively passive (Pavlov 1928). The properties of the nervous system are clearly identified as a predisposing factor in the neurotic disorders.

Unlike Pavlov, who remained a physiologist in outlook, Watson was not prepared to reduce classical conditioning to brain activity. Indeed, in his book, *Behaviourism* (1930), he implicitly criticises Pavlov as one of those *'Psychologists (who) talk . . . quite voluably about the formation of new pathways in the brain, as though there were a group of tiny servants of Vulcan there who run through the nervous system with hammer and chisel digging new tracks and deepening old ones'.*

But Watson's contribution to abnormal psychology consists largely in his assertion of the importance of learning. The psychologist's task was to discover the ways in which the elemental conditioned reflexes combined to form complex behaviours. He believed that the process of conditioning could account for many of the conflicts and behavioural difficulties found in the mentally ill. Indeed, he also considered that conditioning could lay the foundations for the onset of actual organic changes which could lead finally to infections and lesions (Watson 1930).

One of the oldest beliefs about learning is that our behaviour is determined by its effects. Jeremy Bentham's utilitarian emphasis upon pleasure and pain is one expression of this belief and his ideas were subsequently reflected in several different psychological theories. A restatement of the 'Pleasure principle' can be found for instance in Freudian psycho-analysis.

The second sort of conditioning, *operant conditioning,* has its roots in the work of Thorndike. Thorndike was influenced by the comparative tradition of Romanes and of Lloyd Morgan, who was interested in the possibility that simple associative processes might be found to account for the adaptive learnt behaviour of animals. His book, *Animal Intelligence,* was a landmark in the development of psychology. It described a series of experiments concerned with learning and memory. These experiments used a wooden puzzle-box with an escape door held shut by a catch: this could be released by pulling a loop hanging in the box (or by turning a catch in some models). The cats, when placed in this box, showed various random movements which Thorndike refers to as trial and error behaviour. Eventually the cat accidentally releases itself, and on subsequent occasions there is an irregular but generally progressive decrease in the length of time before the animal makes the correct response. It was on the basis of this work that Thorndike (1911) formulated his law of effect.

The Law of Effect is that: of several responses made to the same situation, those which are accompanied or closely followed by satisfaction to the animal will, other things being equal, be more firmly connected with the situation, so that, when it recurs, they will be more likely to recur; those which are accompanied or closely followed by discomfort to the animal will, other things being equal, have their connections with that situation weakened, so that when it recurs, they will be less likely to recur. The greater the satisfaction or discomfort, the greater the strengthening or weakening of the bond.

Watson was highly critical of what he regarded as the mentalistic language in this formulation, and he argued that Thorndike appeared to 'believe habit formation is implanted by kind fairies' in his suggestion that pleasure stamps in the successful response and displeasure stamps out the unsuccessful one (Watson 1930).

Thorndike was later to modify his views on this question of reward and punishment when it became clear that punishment did not always have the clear-cut effect of stamping out the unsuccessful response. Instead, he began to lay greater stress on the effects of reward in the modification of behaviour (Thorndike 1932). One of the best-known experimental contradictions of the Law of Effect was offered by Muezinger (1934). In a study of the effects of punishment on discrimination learning, one group of experimental animals was rewarded for correct responses and punished for incorrect responses. This led to a more rapid rate of learning than among the group which was merely rewarded for making a correct choice. However, the results also showed that *punishing the correct response* produced a more rapid rate of learning than reward alone. This is clearly contrary to the predictions made by the Law of Effect.

Thorndike modified his views on punishment by suggesting that the effects of both 'satisfiers' and 'annoyers' upon learning were dependent upon what they caused the animal to do. But this modification brings the position back towards an associative learning model. Thorndike suggests that the future response to a situation is best predicted by the past associations; that is, stimuli which act during a response tend to evoke that response on subsequent occasions (Guthrie 1952).

Thorndike's views had a strong influence upon theories of learning and directed them towards the use of reward or reinforcement as a basic concept in learning. His ideas provided a foundation for the work of Hull, Spence, Mowrer, Skinner and, more generally, for those psychologists who reject simple association in favour of the concept of reinforcement. Clark Hull provided a synthesis of Pavlov's work on conditioned reflexes and Thorndike's research on trial and error learning. Hull's hypothetico-deductive theory of behaviour (Hull 1943, 1952) used intervening variables to extend the straightforward stimulus-response model into an S-O-R formula. Two of the most important intervening variables were habit strength (S^HR) and drive (D), and Hull laid particular emphasis on reinforcement as the central principle of learning (Hull 1937). The essence of reinforcement was drive reduction; any response which preceded drive reduction would become associated with that drive. Hull argued that classical conditioning and trial and error learning were both to be explained by this drive reduction principle and not by different principles or laws (Hull 1943).

Another behaviourist of this period was Edward Tolman. Tolman differed from most of his colleagues in his interest in behaviour at the molar rather than the molecular level and in his emphasis upon the purposive character of behaviour (Tolman 1948). This introduction of cognitive factors stood in marked contrast to the rather mechanistic formulations of Watson and Pavlov, and in his claim that learning was a process of acquiring knowledge, of learning the meaning of what leads to what, Tolman can be regarded as one of the pioneers of the recent cognitive trend in abnormal psychology. In his attempt to develop a 'purposive behaviourism' he again drew attention to an active, intentional and purposive view of man. A common theme shared by the various cognitive theories is that behaviour is not simply determined by physical input that impinges on the senses, but rather depends upon the selection and transformation of information taken from stimuli.

2. The Neurotic Disorders

*Definitions are a kind of scratching and generally leave a
sore place more sore than before (Samuel Butler).*

2.1 Psychiatric Diagnosis

A medical diagnosis is a definition. The term 'diagnosis' is derived from the Greek and
implies the distinguishing or discernment of a disease. But it implies other things, too.
Without a proper diagnosis in medicine it is impossible to arrive at a rational prognosis
and treatment of the disease (Warner 1952). Similarly, in psychiatry the diagnostic
classification of data is usually expected to go beyond the description of behaviour and to
make a statement about the past, present and future states of the patient (Frank 1975;
Slater and Roth 1974). By medical criteria, this emphasis upon the information that is to
be conveyed by the diagnosis is crucial, and the evaluation of the current diagnostic
system is largely dependent upon its success in this function.

Diagnosis need not be tied to any particular system of classification, though it is usually
identified with the symptomatological classification system derived from Kraeplin. The
system of classification that is used will depend to a large extent upon the theoretical bias
of the person involved. The phrases 'unresolved Oedipal complex' from psycho-analysis,
'manic depression' from orthodox psychiatric classification and 'introverted neurotic'
from trait theory are all diagnostic classifications (Caveny et al. 1955); though it must be
said that they represent very different sorts of diagnoses.

Some critics (notably the phenomenologists and existentialists) have taken the extreme
position of rejecting all systems of classification in psychological medicine. Classification
is seen not only as a useless exercise, but also as a potentially destructive barrier to
therapy (Rogers 1965; Menninger 1948). The terms 'neurosis' and 'psychosis' have been
described as wrong labels with wrong implications which are both obsolete and dangerous (Menninger, Mayman and Pruyser 1963). Anthony Clare (1976) offered a mordant
statement of this position which regards psychiatric classification as:

> an utterly unproductive form of occupational therapy for those psychiatrists who have little
> inclination to delve into the deeper recesses of their patients' minds, less stomach for what they
> might find there, little aptitude for intuitive understanding, and no ability to empathize with or
> imagine themselves into their patients' predicaments. A preoccupation with description and
> classification is itself portrayed as a symptom, an abnormal psychological phenomenon whereby
> psychiatrists defend themselves against their own inadequacy and fear by emphasizing the 'objec-
> tivity' inherent in their arid statistical and classificatory approaches and by hiding behind a
> smokescreen of measurements and 'scientific' jargon.

Jellinek (1939) on the other hand has argued that there is no justification for abandon-
ing classification in psychiatry, but that the system must be more securely based than it
has been in the past. He describes two needs that must be satisfied by classification, the
most important of which is that of organising the data according to 'homologous or

analagous characteristics . . . (which) reflect common origin'. This function of classifying a set of objects or events into subclasses according to certain common characteristics has also been stressed by Hempel (1961); and in psychological medicine it involves the attempt to classify according to common signs, symptoms or other identifying characteristics. An adequate classification of the data is an almost indispensable requirement for the development of theory, although the classification itself depends upon the theory and theoretical assumptions. This latter point is of some significance since it implies that the concept of neurosis itself is dependent upon theoretical assumptions (albeit unstated).

In Kraeplin's classification system there were eight major categories. The system in use between World Wars I and II contained 24 categories, and the 1952 nosology of the American Psychiatric Association had almost 100 diagnoses. The second edition of the Diagnostic and Statistical Manual of Mental Disorders (DSM II 1968) now contains over 100 different diagnostic entities. This system (DSM II) and the World Health Organization's Eighth Edition of the International Classification of Diseases (ICD 8), upon which DSM II is based, represent the two established nosologies of psychiatry. (A third edition of the Diagnostic and Statistical Manual is currently being prepared.) Among the developments that have taken place in the American system (DSM II) is the general elimination of the word 'reaction' as applied to the neuroses. This seems to imply a return to an earlier and more classical Kraeplinian typology (though this was not the intention of the APA Committee on nomenclature and statistics), and the uncertainties surrounding the terminology of diagnosis reflected in this change indicate a fundamental confusion about the nature of the various neurotic disorders (i. e. whether they are to be seen as reactions or conditions). But despite the large number of revisions in the official systems, no truly satisfactory system has emerged (Shakow 1965), and the ever-increasing complexity has not been accompanied by any real advance in the information contained in the diagnostic terms themselves. Howells (1970) commented that

> Developments in a field depend on a number of factors, but probably none so retards progress in psychiatry today as the confusions of its nosology and, linked with it, the lack of agreement on criteria for defining syndromes together with the imprecision of its nomenclature.

It might be said that the neurotic disorders can be approached from different theoretical levels and the failure to take account of this has also tended to obscure many discussions of the neuroses.

There is general agreement upon the need for some sort of classification system (Eysenck 1960c; Maher 1966; Shakow 1965). Unless it is possible to isolate and define a particular disorder or dysfunction, there is little chance of investigating its determinants. But it is equally important to be able to define and measure the symptoms of a given disorder before we attempt any classification, and the widespread devaluation of the importance of symptoms has only further confused this already confused area.

In the most general sense classification systems are devices by which complex material may be reduced to a simpler and more intelligible form through a process of ordering the phenomena according to certain of their similarities. The classes chosen for this purpose are therefore best seen as abstractions imposed from above by the scientist or diagnostician, and not as 'things' inherent in the real world. Nor is there only one system of classification which is appropriate for a given set of phenomena. This depends upon the purposes of the investigator.

In psychiatry there is considerable disagreement about the requirements which should be met by the diagnosis. It has been suggested by psychiatrists who are committed to the organic or medical model that diagnosis in psychiatry should be treated in exactly the same way as in medicine. The disorders included within a particular category (for instance the neuroses) are expected to have characteristics in common, and these characteristics are in turn required to be different from those of other categories, for instance the psychoses (Brill 1967). The psychiatric classification system also assumes that the major clinical variables form distinctive patterns which appear as *qualitatively discrete* and discontinuous disorders (Strauss 1975). Brill (1974) has defended this traditional medical approach to psychiatric classification and lists six requirements of an acceptable clinical classification. One of the points that he raises is that the diagnoses should meet the requirements of validity and reliability. Clearly any adequate system of classification must produce the same result each time it is applied to a specific problem, and it must also measure what it was intended to measure.

These basic requirements of the medical diagnostic system are that the classifications should not be merely descriptive, that the data should be divided into independent and discrete categories, that the classifications should be reliable and that they should be valid. But before going on to examine the adequacy of the psychiatric classification system for the neuroses, it is necessary to describe how neurotic disorders are actually classified. Most sources are in general agreement that anxiety is the chief characteristic of neurosis. Surprisingly, the term 'anxiety' was hardly used in psychology and psychiatry until the late 1930s, and the wide currency that the term now enjoys can be traced back to its introduction by Freud as a translation of *Angst* (Sarbin 1964). The term itself, however, has a deceptive simplicity. It is used by behaviour therapist, psycho-analysts, psychiatrists and physiological psychologists, and its meaning changes each time. Cattell and Scheier (1961) found that there were 120 different procedures used to assess anxiety. There is no single unequivocal definition of anxiety. As an inferred construct with numerous different meanings, the ways in which the term is used will depend upon the theoretical persuasion of the clinician or the experimenter.

The definition of anxiety offered by DSM II reflects the Freudian influence: Anxiety '. . . may be felt and expressed directly, *or it may be controlled unconsciously and automatically by conversion, displacement and various other psychological mechanisms'* (my italics). This comment removes the statement from the realm of description and links it to the inferences and assumptions of a particular model of neurosis. The failure to distinguish between observation and inference has been a common feature of psycho-dynamic thinking and has led to unavoidable tautologies in their theoretical statements.[1]

Apart from laying emphasis upon anxiety as a chief characteristic of the neuroses, DSM II describes the neurotic disorders as causing psychological distress which the person seeks to avoid. The neuroses are also frequently said to differ from the psychoses in the patient's awareness of his own disabilities, his lack of gross distortions of perception and his lack of severe personality disorganisation.

---

1 Ultimately it may be true, as Lakatos (1970) has argued, that there is no clear division between observational and theoretical propositions. Nonetheless, it seems to me to be of considerable importance to distinguish between such statements as 'this condition (hypochondriacal neurosis) is dominated by preoccupation with the body and with fear of presumed diseases of various organs' and 'symptoms (of hysterical neurosis) . . . are symbolic of the underlying conflicts.'

2.2 The Neuroses

2.2.1 Anxiety Neurosis

DSM II describes this neurosis as characterised by anxious over-concern which may extend to panic, and which is frequently associated with somatic symptoms. Unlike phobic neurosis, anxiety may occur under any circumstances, and it is not restricted to particular situations, objects or events. It is necessary to distinguish this neurosis from normal states of apprehension and fear which occur in realistically dangerous situations.

Individuals with anxiety neurosis may be thought of as experiencing directly the discomfort and distress generated by that anxiety, whereas other neurotics have developed methods of redirecting the anxiety into certain symptoms which relieve the immediate distress (Mackay 1975). Those who suffer from 'free-floating anxiety' tend to experience a persistent tension, though this may occasionally be interrupted by acute crises in the form of panic attacks.

2.2.2 Hysterical Neurosis

The psycho-dynamic model has also had an influence upon the formulation offered for the hysterical reactions.

'This neurosis is characterized by an involuntary psychogenic loss or disorder of function. Symptoms characteristically begin and end suddenly in emotionally charged situations and are symbolic of the underlying conflicts. Often they can be modified by suggestion alone' (DSM II).

The suggestion that symptoms are *symbolic* and that they imply the existence of *underlying conflicts* (presumably in a causal role) may be seen as a further commitment of psychiatry to the psycho-dynamic position. In more general terms these comments show the subtle interrelationship between concepts and theoretical assumptions.

2.2.3 Hysterical Neurosis, Conversion and Dissociative Types

In conversion, the special senses and voluntary nervous system are affected, and the symptoms may take the form of blindness, deafness, anaesthesias, paraesthesias, paralysis, ataxias and sometimes seizures of a pseudo-epileptiform character. The pseudo-neurological symptoms in particular tend to correspond to the lay notions of such disorders and are not based upon the anatomical organisation. They are frequently variable and may dramatically disappear without apparent reason. The patient may show an inappropriate lack of concern about his symptoms, and it is often found that these provide secondary gains through winning the patient the sympathy of others, or by relieving them of some unpleasant responsibility. DSM II warns that the conversion type of hysterical neurosis must be distinguished from physiological disorders which are mediated by the autonomic nervous system, presumably on the grounds that these are not under voluntary control, though this assumption may not be warranted (Miller 1969; Kamiya 1969), and also from malingering which is done consciously.

It is worth drawing attention to the phrase 'secondary gains' in this statement. If it is accepted as a *definition,* then it clearly carries a certain theoretical bias. The clear implication is that the conversion neurosis is caused by factors other than the social rewards associated with it. Operant learning theorists might well object to this presupposition.

In dissociative neuroses, alterations may occur in the patient's state of consciousness or in his identity, to produce such symptoms as amnesia, somnambulism, fugue and multiple personality (DSM II).

2.2.4 Phobic Neurosis

The phobic neurosis is characterised by intense fear or dread of an object, event or situation which the patient consciously recognises as presenting no real danger to him. The apprehension may be experienced as fatigue, faintness, palpitations, sweating, nausea and panic. DSM II includes within its definition of phobic neurosis certain psycho-dynamic assumptions. The phobias are described as being attributed to fears which have been displaced onto the phobic object from some other object of which the patient is unaware. Many clinicians working within a behaviour therapy framework might wish to dissociate themselves from this implication of the symbolic significance of phobic fears.

2.2.5 Obsessive-Compulsive Neurosis

This disorder is characterised by the persistent intrusion of unwanted thoughts, urges or actions that the patient feels he cannot control or prevent. The thoughts may consist of single words or ideas, or more often they may be trains of thought. These may or may not be nonsensical. The attempt to dispel these experiences may lead to an inner struggle which occupies all the person's concentration, and there can also be severe anxiety when obsessive-compulsive activities are interfered with. The actions vary from simple movements to complex rituals such as compulsive repeated handwashing, and they are often bizarre or eccentric. Sometimes the actions are seen as a means of warding off the threat associated with morbid thoughts. Obsessive-compulsive phenomena are sometimes found in endogenous depression, schizophrenia and some organic states (notably encephalitis), and ICD-8 states that such instances should be excluded from this neurotic category.

2.2.6 Depressive Neurosis (Reactive Depression)

In reactive depression the extreme dejection is seen as a response to some stressful event or series of difficulties. DSM II again includes certain unnecessary assumptions about the significance of internal conflicts in its definition. Reactive depression has usually been distinguished from psychotic, endogenous depressive illness. ICD-8, for instance, notes that symptoms which are usually found in affective psychosis, such as early-morning waking, loss of weight, self-depreciation and marked retardation, are not typically found in this state, though the distinction between the two conditions is far from clear (Kendell 1975).

2.2.7 Neurasthenic Neurosis (Neurasthenia)

This condition is characterised by complaints of chronic weakness, easy fatigability and, sometimes, exhaustion. Unlike hysterical neurosis, the patient's complaints are genuinely distressing to him and there is no evidence of secondary gain (DSM II).

Despite the agreement of DSM II and ICD-8 upon this neurotic disorder, it is one of the most vague categories. DSM II suggests that it be differentiated from anxiety neurosis by the nature of the predominant complaint and from reactive depression by the moderation of the depressive symptoms. The earlier DSM I referred to this condition as a psychophysiological nervous system reaction. A further complication is that such neurotic states are virtually identical to the separate diagnosis of asthenic personality (included within the personality disorder category). This behaviour pattern is characterised by easy fatigability, low energy level, lack of enthusiasm, marked incapacity for enjoyment and over-sensitivity to physical and emotional stress (DSM II). DSM II also adds the instruction 'this disorder must be differentiated from "Neurasthenic Neurosis"', but no assistance is given to the diagnostician as to how this might be achieved. Apart from illustrating a further weakness inherent in the psychiatric nosology, the vagueness of the definitions offered for neurasthenic neurosis raises the doubt as to the value of maintaining a separate diagnostic term for this disorder.

2.2.8 Hypochondriacal Neurosis
In this condition, the patient shows a persistent anxious preoccupation with his health, often in the form of a fear of presumed diseases of various organs. The fears do not achieve the same degree of intensity that is sometimes found in the delusions of psychotic depression, but they persist despite reassurance or contrary evidence. Unlike hysterical neurosis, there are no actual losses or distortions of function.

2.2.9 Depersonalisation Neurosis (Depersonalisation Syndrome)
This syndrome is dominated by feelings of unreality and of estrangement from the self, body or surroundings – by an unpleasant feeling of strangeness or unreality. Sometimes the person feels that his own actions have an automatic, robot-like quality.

2.2.10 Other Neuroses
This classification includes specific psycho-neurotic disorders that are not described elsewhere. DSM II mentions 'writer's cramp' as an example and warns the clinician against using this category for patients who present with 'mixed neuroses', which it suggests should be diagnosed according to their predominant symptom.

2.3 Problems of Diagnosis

The foregoing categories may be used as an initial statement of the different sorts of neurotic disorders, but there are, necessarily, disagreements about the specific expressions of neurosis. This is partly due to the different theoretical assumptions made by different authors. Although they are not explicitly included in the above categories, the following disorders have also been regarded as neuroses: tics, stuttering, enuresis, various psychosomatic disorders such as asthma, headaches dermatitis, insomnia, obesity, alcoholism and drug dependence. At the other extreme, some psycho-analysts have placed great emphasis upon the concept of character neurosis which may be found in the absence of specific symptoms.

At the time of writing this book, the second edition of the Diagnostic and Statistical Manual is being revised, and it seems likely that DSM III will dispense completely with the general category of 'neurosis'. The various neurotic disorders will instead be reclassified under other headings. Neurotic depression, for instance, is to be subsumed under 'affective disorders'; phobias, obsessional and compulsive disorders, and generalised anxiety disorders are each included within the 'anxiety disorders' section; hysterical and conversion neuroses appear under 'somatoform disorders', and depersonalisation neurosis is included in the 'dissociative disorders' category.[2] The traditional category of

---

2 This is taken from the draft of Axes I and II of DSM III, available from January 16 1978.

'neurasthenic neurosis', which was included in DSM II and ICD 8, has been omitted from the revised American system (which may not be a bad thing in view of its vagueness).

But apart from abolishing the general category of 'neurosis', DSM III remains very much a part of the psychiatric-medical tradition. If the specific diagnoses are required to go beyond description and to make a statement of aetiology and prognosis (Warner 1952; Kendell 1975; Slater and Roth 1974), then the psychiatric nosology must be regarded as a failure, since apart from a few psycho-dynamic assumptions about the causes of neurotic disorders, the diagnoses are largely descriptive.

After a comprehensive survey of the research concerning psychiatric diagnoses, Frank (1975) concludes that the evidence weighs heavily against the current system of classification used in psychiatry: the system is purely descriptive, and Frank argues that to be useful, the diagnostic statements should provide information about the individual beyond merely describing his symptoms. However, Frank is probably assuming that a classification system of this sort could *in principle* be built upon symptomatology. This is doubtful, since invariant conjunctions of symptoms are not to be expected in psychiatric disorders, and it is the persistent assumption that there is some deeper disease entity which underlies the symptom which has again produced this breakdown in the system. By asserting that the diagnoses are 'purely descriptive', Frank overstates his case. Paradoxically, a purely descriptive system could be of more value than the present one, in which diagnostic statements based upon aetiology alternate with others based upon symptom description. Zubin (1967) has complained about the puzzling failure of diagnoses to match with symptoms in a system which is largely based upon overt symptomatology. This failure is largely a result of the confusing mixture of aetiological and descriptive content of the diagnoses themselves. The simultaneous use of these two different approaches in diagnosis increases the chaos in psychiatric classification, and Essen-Möller (1967) has advocated the complete separation of these aspects. Given the present state of knowledge (or ignorance) concerning most psychiatric disorders, disagreements over aetiology are inevitable. The function of science is both to describe and to explain events, and a descriptive system which avoided unnecessary assumptions about aetiology could be useful in its delineation and clarification of the problem to be explained.

The present system has other failings which are also due to the inclusion of alternate statements of symptom description and aetiology in the diagnoses. It is not clear, for instance, whether or not more than one diagnosis should be made. It is a fundamental principle of most classification systems and a traditional aspiration of all branches of medicine that each patient should be restricted to membership of a single diagnostic category (Kendell 1975).

In DSM I, certain multiple diagnoses were forbidden (e. g. alcoholism could not be made as a separate diagnosis when it was associated with an *underlying* disorder). The special instructions for DSM II, on the other hand, state that multiple diagnoses are permissible and cite as an example the fact that a patient with anxiety neurosis may develop morphine addiction. But this example avoids the fundamental problem inherent in multiple diagnosis. There are fewer difficulties raised by the use of multiple diagnoses for different categories of disorders (such as neuroses and drug dependence) than by the use of multiple diagnoses *within* a category.

Jaspers (1972) considered the difficulties raised by this problem and proposed a diagnostic hierarchy in which his Group I disorders took precedence over Group II disorders; these in turn took precedence over Group III disorders. Nonetheless, Jaspers recognised that his proposal was unsatisfactory, particularly for the neuroses and personality disorders, and suggested that the use of categorical diagnoses might have to be abandoned for a classification system in which every case may appear as often as the diagnostician likes. Within such a system, 'all the possible kinds of data can be enumerated but we are no longer enumerating diseases'.

More recently, Foulds restated the hierarchical principle. He suggested four classes of personal illness – class 4, delusions of disintegration; class 3, integrated delusions (e. g. of grandeur or persecution); class 2, neurotic symptoms (conversion, dissociative, phobic, compulsive and ruminative symptoms); and class 1, dysthymic states (anxiety and depression) (Foulds and Bedford 1975). All members of class 4 should also fall into classes 3, 2 and 1; members of class 3, into classes 2 and 1, and members of class 2, also into class 1. It is interesting that Foulds proposed the separation of anxiety and depression from the other neurotic disorders on the grounds that the relationship between anxiety and depression and the conversion, dissociative, phobic, compulsive and ruminative symptoms is different from that between pairs of these symptom groups (Foulds and Bedford 1976). For this reason, anxiety and depression were allotted a lower position in the hierarchy.

Lesse (1970) used a similar hierarchical model in his study of the psychosomatic disorders. Of 151 patients suffering from autonomic faciocephalagia (cluster headaches), migraine headaches, essential hypertension, colitis, asthma and neurodermatitis, Lesse found that psychosomatic disorders rarely exist as an isolated clinical entity. They usually occur as part of a wider neurotic disorder and are usually secondary to anxiety. Such other symptoms as phobias, hypochondriasis, obsessions and compulsions were generally noted prior to the appearance of psychosomatic problems.

Another problem for the clinician who wishes to make a single differential diagnosis is that in practice, anxiety and depression are often found together. One extensive study of depression (Grinker et al. 1961) found five factors underlying diagnosed depressive disorders. These were (a) hopelessness, sadness, helplessness and feelings of unworthiness; (b) a concern over material loss and conviction that the emotional state could be remedied by external changes; (c) guilt over some perceived wrongdoing and a wish to make restitution; (d) envy, loneliness, martyred affliction and secondary gains through provoking guilt in others; and (e) a free-floating anxiety factor. Grinker's investigation showed that the anxiety factor was an important part of the clinical concept of depression. A diagnosis of depression was contingent not only upon depressed affect in the patient, but also on the presence of anxiety; and in those cases in which there was only minimal depressive affect, the anxiety factor greatly increased the probability of a 'depressed' diagnosis. The instructions of DSM II that the diagnostician 'should not lose sight of the rule of parsimony and diagnose more conditions than are necessary to account for the clinical picture' is unhelpful here. If each of the different neurotic disorders are important features of the patient's difficulties, the psychiatrist can only list them all or limit himself, on the basis of a subjective choice, to a single 'differential diagnosis'. Masserman and Carmichael (1938) have complained about a similar problem. One hundred patients who had been admitted to the psychiatry department of the University of Chicago Clinic were re-examined after 1 year. Except for those individuals who showed a 'well-demarcated anxiety syndrome', there was a wide variation in the diagnostic categories, 'indicating the mixed character of nearly all neurotic and psychotic reactions'.

The tendency for mixed states to occur poses another major problem for any system such as that of Kraeplin which relies upon categorical distinctions between the disorders

(Curran et al., 1972). The same difficulty arises in those cases in which the overt symptomatology changes over time. In other areas of psychiatry the problem is even worse. In drug addiction, for instance, the use of discrete categories for dependence upon opiates, barbiturates, stimulants, hallucinogens or other drugs breaks down completely, since the general pattern of drug taking is that of multiple drug abuse (Blumberg et al. 1974; Gossop and Connell 1975; Gossop 1978 a). The diligent diagnostician must resolve the mutually exclusive requirements of validity and of parsimony for himself; the system has broken down.

A further difficulty arises if the diagnostician chooses to select from a large number of potential diagnoses in order to present his own interpretation of the most salient features; but despite the problems inherent in this introduction of subjective bias, this is exactly what the psychiatrist is instructed to do. DSM II states that for patients with several different neurotic disorders, the clinician should make a diagnosis according to the predominant symptom. The simplicity of the word 'predominant' has little in common with the complexity of the selective perceptual and judgmental processes involved in the actual choice of what constitutes a 'predominant symptom'. This introduction of subjectivity could be confidently predicted to lower the inter-rater reliability of the system.

2.4 Reliability and Consistency

Kreitman (1961) stressed the importance of reliability, since no set of observations can be adequately incorporated within a body of knowledge unless they meet the basic requirements of reliability. In the case of psychiatric diagnosis, reliability can be defined either as the amount of agreement between different observers when examining the same subjects, or as the agreement between an initial and a subsequent diagnosis. Zubin (1967) refers to the former as 'agreement' and the latter as 'consistency'. Hunt et al. (1953) looked at the consistency of diagnoses over time and found that the average agreement between psychiatrists on major categories (psychosis, neurosis, etc.) was only 54%; and for specific diagnoses within categories, the average agreement was 33%. For the neuroses the problem was even worse. Only 24% of the category diagnoses of neurosis were in agreement, and for specific neurotic disorders only 12% agreement was achieved. One of the largest studies of diagnostic reliability was conducted by Norris (1959), who reported the results of an investigation of over 6000 patients. The reliability of the category diagnoses for various disorders between occasions were: functional psychoses, 89%; neurosis, 46%; and character disorder, 34%. No figures were given for agreement levels achieved in the specific diagnoses of neurotic disorders.

In an investigation of the amount of agreement between raters, Kreitman et al. (1961) reported 52% agreement for the general diagnosis of neurosis and 28% for specific diagnoses. Similar results are presented by Ash (1949), Beck (1962) and Kaelbling and Volpe (1963).

Zubin (1967) has reviewed the evidence for the reliability of diagnoses, and states that the level of agreement for the neuroses is low and variable. For the diagnosis of an unspecified neurosis, the agreement varies between 16% and 56%, for reactive depression between 18% and 63% and for anxiety states between 27% and 55%. Schmidt and Fonda (1956) concluded that some diagnoses reached satisfactory levels of reliability; on the diagnoses of schizophrenia, for instance, the agreement level was between 73% and

95%, but they point to the unreliability of diagnoses on the personality disorders and the neuroses, where agreement between psychiatrists was almost completely absent. *These overall levels of agreement and consistency are far too low for individual diagnoses of neurotic disorders to be accepted as reliable.*

The findings of Kreitman et al. (1961) suggest that the fault lies with the system itself, and not with the psychiatrists. In their study they compared the agreement between the psychiatrists on duration of illness, family history, previous illness, symptomatology and other variables. On none of these were there significant inter-rater differences, and the authors conclude that the low reliabilities were not therefore due to differences in the application of diagnoses between psychiatrists. Ward et al. (1962) investigated the sources of disagreement in diagnosis, and noted nine basic problems. The most profound source of error was due to the nosological system itself (62.5%), though they also attribute 32.5% of the variance to the inconstant behaviour of the diagnostician. Only 5% of the variance could be attributed to the inconstant behaviour of the patient. Much of this unreliability is probably directly due to the confusion between descriptive and explanatory statements that are contained in the diagnostic system.

Wing and his colleagues (1974) have taken these objections to the psychiatric system of diagnosis more seriously than most, though they still believe that 'psychiatric disease theories can be useful in everyday clinical practice'. The Present State Examination, a structured interview, was devised by these workers as an attempt to improve the reliability and validity of diagnoses, and a similar effort has been made by Goldberg (1972) with the General Health Questionnaire.

2.5 Validity

The whole problem of validity in this context is extremely complex, since there is no ultimate criterion against which the diagnoses or measures can be validated.

Everitt et al. (1971) reported a sophisticated attempt to validate the traditional psychiatric system of classification using cluster analysis on data derived from 250 English and 250 American patients. A total of 728 items of information was available for each patient. The authors found that three distinct categories emerged as relatively distinct clusters. These were the manic phase of manic depression, paranoid schizophrenia and psychotic depression. A fourth category, schizophrenia, was also found to present a fairly distinct cluster. But in the case of the neurotic disorders, there was a striking failure to find any sort of cluster. This failure was particularly significant for neurotic depression, since there were more than 60 patients with this diagnosis in the two series. A similar failure to obtain any neurotic cluster has also been reported by Pilowsky et al. (1969).

However, other studies by Derogatis and his colleagues suggest that the conventional descriptions of the neurotic disorders may have some validity (Derogatis et al. 1970, 1971a, 1971b; Williams et al. 1968). These studies found a high coincidence between five clinical clusters for the neurotic disorders and the results of factor analyses. Using large numbers of neurotic out-patients, all of whom displayed anxiety, they found factors of:
1) *Somatisation.* This was characterised by feelings of heaviness in the limbs, numbness in parts of the body, muscular soreness, weakness and pains in the chest.

2) *Obsessive-Compulsive-Phobic.* The items that showed strong positive loadings for this factor were having to check and re-check actions, difficulty in remembering things, difficulty in making decisions, difficulty in concentrating and worries about carelessness.
3) *Irritability-Over-sensitivity.* This factor loaded on items such as feeling easily annoyed by things and critical of others, outbursts of temper, feelings easily hurt and feelings of inferiority.
4) *Depression.* This was characterised by thoughts of ending one's life, loss of sexual interest and pleasure, general depressive mood and hopelessness about the future.
5) *Anxiety.* The anxiety items included feeling fearful, sensations of nervousness or shakiness, suddenly feeling frightened for no obvious reason, sensations of one's heart pounding and feeling tense or keyed-up.

Although these findings cannot be freely generalised beyond anxious neurotic patients, the results provide some support for the validity of the descriptive classification of the neurotic disorders. Derogatis et al. (1970, 1971 a, 1971 b) suggest that the factors may represent primary or 'core' dimensions of the neurotic disorders.

These results and those of Everitt et al. (1971) suggest that the neurotic disorders appear to merge into one another, and that no independent *types* of neurotic patients can be distinguished. However, there is some evidence to support the validity of the neurotic disorders as describing separate dimensions which underlie the *symptoms* and manifestations of neurotic psychopathology.

The evidence that has been presented suggests that the traditional system of classification is extremely unreliable and inconsistent in its application to the neurotic disorders. This is probably due to the confounding of the descriptive and explanatory functions of the diagnoses themselves; and it has been suggested that purely descriptive statements of the nature of the neurotic disorders would at least have the advantage of increasing the level of agreement upon what is to constitute the *explicandum*. The studies of Derogatis and his colleagues provide some support for the validity of the traditional clinical descriptions of the neuroses. A further problem with the current psychiatric system is its use of a categorical system to describe the neurotic disorders. Hine and Williams (1975) reach the same conclusion about the inadequacy of this system of classification and propose that it should be replaced by a dimensional system. As Hempel (1961) has pointed out, most sciences start out with a typology based upon dichotomies, but frequently move on to continuous, dimensional systems.

2.6 Social Context

Another reason for rejecting the categorical, disease-entity notion is that the social context within which both patient and clinician operate has a profound influence upon the diagnostic process and upon the neurotic disorder itself. Sandifer et al. (1969) presented a description of the psychopathology of a group of patients to 41 psychiatrists in England and America. In their evaluation of the clinical material, the most striking finding was that the psychiatrists of the United States reported almost twice as many symptoms as those of the United Kingdom.

Meehl (1973), who is committed both to the notion of disease entities in functional psychiatry and to the Kraeplinian nomenclature as the best system of classification, has implied that diagnoses are unreliable partly because of the 'careless and unskilled' approach of some psychiatrists. The same sort of argument in defence of psychiatric diagnosis has been used by Clare (1976) in reply to the findings presented by Rosenhan.

In his study, Rosenhan (1973) poses the basic question, 'How do we recognise insanity?'

> Do the salient characteristics that lead to diagnoses reside in the patients themselves or in the environments and contexts in which observers find them? From Bleuler, through Kretchmer, through the formulaters of the recently revised Diagnostic and Statistical Manual of the American Psychiatric Association the belief has been strong that patients present symptoms, that the symptoms can be categorised, and, implicitly, that the sane are distinguishable from the insane.

Eight 'normal' volunteers presented at 12 different psychiatric hospitals, complaining that they had been hearing voices which spoke meaningless words such as 'hollow' and 'empty'. These symptoms were chosen because of their similarity to existential symptoms and because of the absence of any reported existential psychosis in the literature. Apart from this single symptom, and the use of a false name and occupation, all other characteristics were presented truthfully from the person's life history, and immediately upon admission to a psychiatric ward, the pseudo-patient ceased to simulate any symptom of abnormality. All but one of the individuals was admitted with a diagnosis of schizophrenia, and discharged as schizophrenic 'in remission' (that is, not as 'cured' or 'normal'); the one patient not diagnosed as schizophrenic was diagnosed as manic depressive. Despite the fact that 35 out of 118 patients voiced their suspicions that the pseudo-patients were only faking, no psychiatrist or any member of staff detected this.

Both Clare (1976) and Wing (1973) take the position that this failure reflects the ill-informed and slipshod approach of the diagnosticians, rather than any weakness inherent in the system itself. It is interesting that this was the same excuse offered by a research and teaching hospital in Rosenhan's report. Subsequently, this institution was informed that one or more pseudo-patients would attempt to gain admission to the hospital over the following 3 months. Since a certain amount of prestige and professional acumen were at stake, the psychiatrists and staff involved could be expected to be more alert to the subtleties of symptomatology. And indeed they were. They were confident that they had detected 41 pseudo-patients (19 of whom were detected both by a psychiatrist and one other staff member). Unfortunately, no pseudo-patient presented himself to the hospital during this period.

The full implications of this disturbing study are far from clear. The results do, however, point to the way that the meaning of behaviour depends upon the context in which it occurs. It should, by now, be common knowledge that perceptions are not passive, accurate representations of the real world, but are highly selective. The Gestalt school showed how important the context was in its effect upon perception, and Sherif (1936) described how our experience is organised around, and modified by, the social circumstances within which it occurs. Other studies have pointed to the distortions in person perception that are dependent upon the psychological state of the perceiver. Kelley (1950), for instance, showed how sensitive person perception can be to subtle verbal cues which are interpreted in terms of the perceiver's implicit personality theory. The meaning of the social interaction and the roles of the individuals involved are also potent influences upon the final perception (Kelley 1948), a finding which has special relevance for the diagnostician. Katz et al. (1969) locked at the diagnostic disagreement among clinicians and suggested that this may be due in part to differences in perception between the observers.

There can be little doubt that the current psychiatric classification system is inadequate. In its defence, Foulds (1955) has argued that its inadequacy does not prove its unsuitability, and that in any case, it should not be replaced until a better substitute is available. This chapter presents the case that a system which was based upon overt symptomatology would have several advantages over the confused psychiatric nosology. In particular, it would improve the chances of agreement between clinicians on the nature of the neurotic disorders, and it would avoid the inappropriate mixture of description and theory that has bedevilled most of the previous work in this area (see also Essen-Möller 1967; and Costello 1970).

3. Neurosis, Normality and Psychosis

3.1 Normality and Abnormality

There has been little explicit discussion of what constitutes mental health, and although it is impossible to practise psychiatry or clinical psychology without some (usually implicit and unstated) concept or assumptions about normality, few clinicians seem to have had either the time or the inclination to give serious consideration to the concept of normality that underlies their work. In order to recognise abnormality we must have some notion of normality. The concept of normality is what philosophers would call *parasitic;* that is, it is dependent upon the existence of some distinction between normality and abnormality. But any attempt to specify what is meant by these terms leads immediately to considerable difficulties, and Aubrey Lewis has described the concept of mental health as 'invincibly obscure' (Lewis 1958).

In the first place, the problem of psychological health or normality is closely related to that of the classification of mental disorders. The traditional medical psychiatric approach usually shows little interest in the question of normality per se and focuses instead upon the specific disease entities (Barton 1959). Mental health is defined in terms of the absence of any clear psychopathology. The influence of this tradition can be seen in the omission of any discussion of the problem of normality from most psychiatric text books (e. g. Slater and Roth 1969; Henderson and Batchelor 1962), though Arieti's *Handbook of American Psychiatry* includes a chapter by Offer and Sabshin (1974). The largely implicit psychiatric concept of normality appears to regard health as an almost universal phenomenon, and one which is characterised by reasonable, rather than ideal, levels of functioning. It is not clear whether the neurotic pathology that differentiates health from illness is the overt symptomatology or some underlying personality factor. As has been described, the diagnostic manuals tend to confuse elements of both in their description of the neuroses, and this further compounds the problem, since the criteria for recognising behavioural symptomatology are very different from those used to identify features of personality. Martin Roth doubts whether the concept of disease can be defined other than in the broadest of terms in either psychiatry or in medicine. This leaves an indistinct line of demarcation between health and disease, but it may still be preferable to the spurious precision to be gained by definition in terms of lesions (Roth 1963). In the absence of any clear discussion of this problem from the medical-psychiatric perspective, the precise relationship between neurosis and health remains unclear.

To the psycho-analyst, freedom from symptoms is not an acceptable criterion of mental health, and psycho-analysts would also reject any definition based upon 'absence of pathology'. Plaut (1960) has even suggested that under some circumstances an absence of symptoms may indicate 'sterility and stagnation'. In psycho-analysis, 'health' and 'sickness' are used as attributes of *individuals* and not of behaviours (Hartmann 1960). Psychologists and psychiatrists with interests in learning theory and behaviour modification, on the other hand, have tended to restrict the use of such terms as 'normal', 'healthy' and 'abnormal' to behaviour or to specific events.

The psycho-analysts, and in particular the Freudian psycho-analysts, have used a concept of normality which is based upon the notion of an unattainable optimal or ideal level of functioning. Offer and Sabshin (1967) traced this position back to Sigmund Freud, whose theory assumed the universality of unconscious conflicts, the Oedipus complex, childhood repression and so forth (Freud 1900, 1905). Freud stated that everyone is to some extent neurotic and that a normal ego, like normality in general, is an ideal fiction (Freud 1901, 1937). Levine (1942) has also suggested that normality is 'non-existent in a complete form', and can only be found 'as (a) relative and quantitative approximation'.

For the psycho-analyst, of course, the ideal fiction of normality refers to personality and not to the subjective feelings of the patient or to the absence of overt symptoms. Melanie Klein (1960) has provided one of the more detailed psycho-analytic descriptions of normality, which she sees in terms of personality integration. Complete integration is again seen to be an unattainable ideal. The important features of normality (in Kleinian terms) are emotional maturity, the capacity to deal with conflicting emotions, and strength of character, each of which derives from infantile experiences of gratification and frustration, and the capacity to resolve the conflicts between one's own emotions, and between the intrapsychic and external realities. Ernest Jones (1950) has been one of the few psycho-analysts to emphasise the importance of social adjustment in any definition of normality, and he includes among his criteria of normality the personal satisfaction of the individual and his effectiveness in social and psychological functioning. The behaviour of the normal person should be both personally satisfying and socially appropriate.

The influence of the psycho-analytic concept of 'normality as ideal' extends beyond psycho-analysis into psychiatry and psychology. Maslow's notions about self-actualisation rely in large measure upon Freudian ideas of normality. Maslow and Mittelmann (1951) suggest that psychological normality consists of adequate self-knowledge, integrated personality, ability to learn from experience and other similar criteria. The self-actualised or ideally normal person emerges as spontaneous, creative, with a sense of humour and aware of, and accepting, both his own needs and those of others. Jahoda (1958) reviewed the literature on mental health and provided a similar description of the constituents of positive mental health. Like Maslow and Klein, Jahoda emphasises the independence, growth and integration of the individual as well as the importance of self-attitudes. But despite the superficial plausibility of this approach to normality as ideal, there are many problems involved in such definitions. In particular the specification of what is to count as 'adequate', 'integrated', 'mature' or 'creative' depends upon culture-bound and value-laden judgments, and these difficulties have not been discussed satisfactorily by the proponents of this perspective. Lewis (1958) referred dismissively to such definitions as a 'clutter of words'. Nor do these lists of the supposed characteristics of normality match the subtle ways in which the concept is actually used.

Unlike the medical perspective, which is usually based upon a categorical system, this concept of 'normality as ideal' relies upon a straight-line continuum between normality and abnormality. Menninger, Mayman and Pruyser (1963) proposed that specific classifications of psychological disorders should be abandoned in favour of a unidimensional system in which the different manifestations of mental illness were to be seen as sequential stages of a single process. This, however, is a rather extreme position. Goldberg (1972) suggested that the distribution of psychiatric symptoms in the general population does not correspond to any dichotomy between 'cases' and 'normals', and that non-psychotic disorders are best seen as being evenly distributed throughout the population. This single dimension varies between 'severe disorder to a hypothetical normality, with many steps between these end-points'.

A more statistically sophisticated notion of normality uses the normal distribution curve as its basis. In this model, 'normal' refers to the middle range of the curve, and both extremes represent the statistically abnormal; that is, they are abnormal because of their infrequency. Offer and Sabshin (1966) discussed this perspective and noted that there are thousands of biochemical tests which are based upon this principle. The statistical perspective is also widely used in the field of psychometrics.

It is one of the more important implications of dimensional approaches to neurosis that no clear dividing line can be drawn between states of mental health and those of neurosis. Many clinical psychologists have been at pains to stress that in its development, its maintenance and in the ways in which it may be altered, abnormal behaviour is no different from normal behaviour. There is no intrinsic difference between the two. The difference is to be found in the reactions of others (Ullmann and Krasner 1967). Accordingly, it is more productive to examine the ways in which a person develops any belief or behaviour pattern rather than how he develops a false belief or a maladaptive pattern of behaviour, since the principles underlying both are the same. Ullmann and Krasner's *Psychological Approach to Abnormal Behaviour (1969)* expressed this position which rejects the distinction between normality and abnormality as *categories.* Indeed, Ullmann and Krasner suggest that the failure to arrive at any single clear definition of abnormality is one of the strongest reasons for attempting to discuss in terms of normality those behaviours that have traditionally been accepted as the subject matter of abnormal psychology. To this extent, the dimensional perspective is often used in a descriptive way as an attempt to avoid the use of such evaluative terms as 'normality'.

Among the strongest advocates of the dimensional approach has been Hans Eysenck (1947a, 1961, 1967). Instead of using a variable number of disease entities which differ from psychiatrist to psychiatrist, Eysenck proposed the use of three dimensions (introversion/extraversion, neuroticism and psychoticism), along which any person may be ranged and given a numerical score. The neuroticism and psychoticism factors (N and P) are the two main independent factors in psychological medicine. Both define continua which range between extreme disorder and normality, and there are no breaks or qualitative differences which make it possible to classify people into separate groups (Eysenck 1961). The psychiatric diagnoses appear not as categories but as points of intersection within the dimensional framework; a diagnosis represents a specific region in multifactor space (Eysenck 1970a). Patients who also fit into that region would have certain resemblances because of their similar position on the relevant dimensions, but these would shade imperceptibly into other diagnoses.

Another personality theorist who has used this dimensional approach is Cattell. Unlike Eysenck, who proposes a single neuroticism factor, Cattell's interpretation of neurosis is multifactorial. Cattell suggests that this approach has its parallels in physical medicine which is in transition from single-cause thinking to a multifactorial view of disease as a dysfunction of the whole organism (Cattell and Scheier 1961). There is an equal emphasis upon the need to relate this quantative approach to personality description to a quantitative description of environmental factors, and Cattell (1957) has suggested a mathematical model for the typing and measurement of environmental events.

A purely statistical interpretation of normality still fails to avoid the pitfalls of value-judgements, which seem to obtrude themselves into any classificatory system. A dimensional system which relies upon the normal distribution of scores faces problems of evaluation concerned with the tails of the curve. It is difficult to think of genius as being abnormal in the same way as idiocy, nor do we think of the extremely well-adjusted and emotionally stable in the same terms as the maladjusted and disturbed person. At the same time this model is not entirely satisfactory in its equation of normality with the middle range of the distribution. This tends to regard conformity to group norms as normality.

On the other hand, a few psychiatrists and psycho-analysts have taken a hard-line, absolutist view of normality. Money-Kyrle (1957), for instance, dismisses the problems of value-judgements and cultural relativity and lays stress upon insight as the crucial factor. This sort of view, however, has few supporters and most writers have been troubled by this problem of value-judgment. Jahoda (1958) has been one of the few psychologists to face up to the problem of values, and she explicitly identified some of the culture-bound values that have influenced concepts of normality (such as the positive evaluation of personal independence and autonomy). Ultimately it seems unlikely that any adequate definition of normality will be achieved which completely avoids this particular difficulty, and the best that can be hoped for is that the value judgements underlying clinical concepts of normality should be explicitly identified.

Goldberg (1972) suggested that a quantitative dimensional measure of psychiatric disturbance provides a *probability estimate* of that person's being a psychiatric case. Goldberg is caught in the dilemma of wishing to use a dimensional as well as a categorical approach; instead of using a simple typology, he argued that some threshold point on the continuum could be chosen to differentiate 'cases' from 'normals'. This faces the same theoretical difficulties as a typological model of abnormality. There can be no clear dividing line. Equally, the assumption that the severity of a psychological disorder can be defined entirely in terms of the phenomena of psychiatric illness faces a number of problems. Minor psychological symptoms are widely distributed in the general population, but the meaning of those symptoms is dependent upon how the individual sees, evaluates and acts upon them, how others act upon them, and in what sort of social situation they occur. It is probably true to say that these aspects of abnormal psychology have been better appreciated by social psychologists and sociologists than by clinical psychologists and psychiatrists.

In one of the classic experimental studies of the effects of cognition upon emotion, Schachter and Singer (1962) demonstrated that emotional states are the result of an interaction between cognitive and physiological factors. Some subjects were told that they were to be given an injection of a vitamin but were actually given adrenalin, a drug which causes autonomic arousal, increased heart rate, sweating, etc. Having received no explanation for these effects, they provided their own interpretation of their experience, based upon the circumstances in which they found themselves. When the subject was in the company of an angry person they themselves felt anger, and when exposed to euphoric behaviour they felt happy. Those subjects who were correctly informed of the effects of the drug showed least emotional response to the behaviour of the experimental confederate, since they already had an appropriate explanation of their state of arousal. Schachter and Singer argue that the physiological arousal itself is indeterminate, and that the cognition channels arousal into specific emotional states. Similar findings have also been reported by Schachter and Wheeler (1962), and Valins (1966) has shown that the subject's perception of his own state of arousal need not be correct in order to affect the resulting emotion. After subjects had received misleading feedback of their own heart rate when viewing certain photographs of nude females, they described a preference for those photographs over others. Conversely, the individual's emotionality can also be decreased by misattributing his naturally occurring emotions to a non-emotional source (Nisbett and Schachter 1966).

This recent emphasis upon the individual's beliefs about his own behaviour has profound implications for the concepts of health and mental illness. It is necessary, for instance, to re-interpret any division between normality and neurosis in the light of the individual's cognitions, since self-attributions affect a whole range of emotional, attitudinal and behavioural responses. The perception of oneself as 'neurotic' carries implications quite distinct from the 'normal' self-perception, and to that extent it is possible to suggest a discontinuity between normality and neurosis – though not in the way proposed by the medical model.

The attribution theorists emphasise self-perceptions. Sociologists tend to place greater emphasis upon the significance of the perceptions of others. Parsons (1952, 1964) defines both health and illness in social terms. Health is defined as the optimum *capacity* of a person for the effective performance of the roles and tasks for which he has been socialised, and illness is also seen as a socially institutionalised role. Both are defined in terms of the individual's participation within a social system. Parsons has pointed out that it is not possible to regard all illnesses as 'natural phenomena' which merely happen to people, though there are still some who attempt to reduce all illnesses to the physiological and biological level and to look for therapies at that level. Parsons offered a statement of how illness constitutes a social role rather than merely a 'condition', and his formulation of the sick-role has been widely used by medical sociologists. There is also an increasing awareness of the value of this concept among clinicians. Parsons discussed the social implications of the sick-role, and in particular the exemptions from social responsibility that are conferred upon the sick. These privileges and exemptions of the sick-role may themselves become objects of secondary gain which the patient learns to value. However, it is one condition of the legitimisation of illness as deviance that the sick individual recognises the inherent undesirability of his sickness. To the extent that the neurotic individual is seen by others to derive gratification from his position (as is also the case with alcoholics and drug addicts) there exists a considerable tension between accepting or rejecting the validity of the sick-role.

One of the most widely used sociological explanations of how individuals come to occupy the sick-role is the societal reaction theory, or labelling theory. Labelling theory makes a basic distinction between primary and secondary deviance. Primary deviance, the fact of which causes a person to be labelled as deviant in the first place, has been said to have at best only marginal implications for the psychic structure of the individual (Lemert 1967); and secondary deviance consists of the ways in which the individual adapts to the problems created by how others react to his primary deviance. Erikson has emphasised that deviance is not to be seen as a property inherent in certain forms of behaviour, but rather that it represents a property which is conferred upon those forms by society (Erikson 1957).

Societal reaction theorists are therefore primarily interested in the social responses of others, arguing that the self-perceptions of the deviant individual depend upon the image of themselves that they receive through the actions of others. Scheff (1966), who applied labelling theory to mental illness, uses this concept to refer to the occupancy of a social role and not to a state of personal distress, behavioural disorganisation or personality disorder. Mental illness is to be seen as an ascribed status dependent upon factors external to the individual.

The principal weaknesses of the societal reactance theory are that it has failed to consider how neuroses (and mental illnesses in general) develop, and it has exaggerated the amount of secondary deviance produced by treating someone who is mentally ill. Gove (1970) examined the assumptions of labelling theory and found that a person's behaviour determines the expectations of others to a greater extent than the reverse, and that a substantial majority of hospitalised individuals present a considerable psychiatric disturbance quite apart from any secondary deviance associated with their sick-role. Cole and Lejeune (1972) also suggest that individuals who are unable to function adequately in a social setting are likely to be motivated to define themselves as sick in order to legitimise their self-defined failure.

This aspect of social adjustment has important implications for the clinical psychologist, and it has been regarded as a crucial feature of psychological health. Some clinicians have used social training programmes as a technique of therapy. Liberman and Raskin (1971), for instance, were able successfully to treat a case of depression through the modification of social behaviour, and Phillips and Zigler (1961) related social competence to the nature of the psychiatric difficulties experienced by different patients. Similar findings were presented by Libet and Lewinsohn (1973), who found that depressed patients were less socially skilled than other non-depressed individuals, and social-skill deficits can be seen as a major feature of many psychiatric disorders (Hersen and Eisler 1976). Gove (1970) accepts that the expectations and social responses of others may have an important effect, but denies that labelling theory offers a sufficient explanation, because of its neglect of the individual's own attitudes and behaviour.

Many individuals who suffer from neurotic problems remain in the 'normal' population and avoid contact with psychiatrists. To that extent they also avoid the stigma of the 'neurotic' label. It is, however, extremely difficult to make any assessment of the prevalence rates of neurosis in the normal population, since the inclusion of any particular case within the 'neurotic' group will reflect as much about the criteria of the investigator as about the difficulties of the person involved.

Essen-Möller (1956) interviewed 2500 inhabitants of a rural area of Sweden and classified the population on a continuum ranging from definite mental illness through personality abnormality to normality. His estimate of life-time prevalence of various disorders was 1.7% for psychosis and 5.2% for neurosis, with about 35% in the 'normal' range. In a later study of the same population, Hagnell (1959, 1968) used a more extensive interview with more overtly psychiatric content and suggested that the figures were 1.7% for psychoses and 13.1% for neuroses. It is interesting that whereas the psychotic disorders were unaffected by the changes in criteria of abnormality, the estimate of the prevalence of neuroses was more than doubled.

Anthony Ryle (1967) conducted a survey of the prevalence rates of neurosis and emotional disturbance among a group of 112 psychiatrically unselected London families. A large proportion of both the adults and children in this group were found to show 'pathological' symptoms, and Ryle argues that those individuals who seek professional help and advice for their neurotic difficulties represent only a fraction of those with such problems. Unfortunately Ryle fails to make clear what were his notions of neurosis, health and normality in this study, and there are many pitfalls involved in the use of retrospective analysis of general practitioners' records for such information. Ryle does use scores from the Cornell Medical Index as a more objective form of data, but here again, Ryle denies that any useful distinction can be made between neurosis and neuroticism (i. e. between neurotic behaviour and personality predisposition). This may well be a hazardous assumption to make. Whether or not the person who scores highly on measures of neuroticism develops a neurotic disorder will depend upon more than his predisposition. Clearly the degree of environmental stress to which he is exposed will play a crucial role.

These weaknesses raise considerable doubts about Ryle's specific findings, though in his general conclusion he may be correct. Another investigation of 46 medical practices in London, for instance, also suggested that neurotic disorders may constitute a sizeable problem for the general practitioner, and that as many as 14% of his consultations may be concerned with such problems (Shepherd et al. 1966; Shepherd 1973). But although I would not wish to deny the general suggestion in these studies that neurotic difficulties are fairly common in the general population, I would like to draw attention to the theoretical nature of the question. The attempt to reduce this issue of prevalence rates of health and neurosis to an empirical question is misguided.

In their investigation of London medical students, Lucas et al. (1965) fall into this sort of error. They conclude that about one-third of their sample showed psychological symptoms such as anxiety, tension and poor concentration. However, these psychological 'symptoms' were generally directly related to some specific situational stress, such as examinations. To focus upon symptomatology to the exclusion of situational factors in this way shows a fundamental misunderstanding of the nature of neurotic disorders. If it is neurotic to respond to stress with anxiety, then we would all be neurotic, and it is probable that such misunderstandings have led to conclusions such as 'anxiety neurosis is the most frequent disorder of civilised life' (Weiss 1942). It remains one of the unfortunate consequences of the medical perspective that neurotic disorders are seen in terms of identifiable illness to the exclusion of social and cognitive factors, and Shey (1971) has drawn attention to iatrogenic anxiety, a problem that has been largely ignored by physicians because of their 'somatic' orientation.

The idea that neurotic disorders can be seen in terms of their objective severity is misconceived; indeed, it is not clear what we could mean by such a notion as objective severity in this instance. The 'severity' will depend upon the personal distress that the individual suffers as a result of his neurotic behaviour: and the distress itself will in turn depend both upon how the person regards his own behaviour and on how others see his behaviour. If he comes to see his anxiety as a 'normal' response to a stressful situation, he may well be able to cope with his anxiety and the situation quite adequately. If, on the other hand, he or others decide to label the anxiety as 'neurotic' or as 'sick', then quite different consequences will follow. He may firstly approach a doctor, in which case the professional and personal criteria that the doctor uses to differentiate normality from neurosis will determine any reaction to the patient. If the doctor does regard the patient as having a neurotic disorder, then the person may fall into the sick-role that has been described by such sociologists as Parsons.

3.2 Neurosis and Psychosis

There are two fundamental issues to be dealt with here. Firstly, whether it is useful to maintain any distinction between neurosis and psychosis; and if it is, whether they are to be represented by different points on the same continuum, or in terms of separate and independent dimensions. Martin Roth (1963) has described how neurosis and psychosis are usually differentiated in terms of a number of characteristics, none of which is on its own sufficient to produce a reliable and valid distinction. In neurosis, the disorder is generally restricted in its effect upon the individual's functioning; the person retains contact with reality and a certain amount of insight into his difficulties. When used to refer to personality, the term is again used to suggest partial dysfunction in which some facets of personality are unaffected. In addition, the neurotic behaviour can often be seen as an exaggeration of ordinary emotional reactivity. Psychoses, on the other hand, have a more global effect upon the individual's personality. All, or most, aspects of behaviour are affected, and there is usually a dramatic reduction in the person's contact with reality. Taylor (1966) expressed this in terms of insight – that psychotic patients lack insight into the truth or falsity of their idiosyncratic beliefs, whereas neurotics generally do have some insight.

Freud distinguished between neurosis and psychosis in the following way: 'Neurosis is the result of a conflict between the ego and its id, whereas psychosis is the analogous outcome of a similar disturbance in the relations between the ego and the external world' *(Neurosis and Psychosis)*. This brief statement provides an outline of the difference in the genesis of the two disorders. However, Freud insisted that the aetiology of a neurosis and of a psychosis is always the same. It consists in a frustration of primitive childhood wishes, though it depends upon the nature of the intrapsychic solution as to whether the resultant disorder proves to be neurotic or psychotic. If in resolving the conflict the ego retains its dependence on external reality and attempts to overcome the demands of the id, the outcome is neurosis: on the other hand, if the ego is itself overcome by the demands of the id, it loses contact with reality with the consequence that the person becomes psychotic.

Freud repeatedly emphasised the idea that those trends and conflicts that he described were not to be seen as 'causes' of psychological disorders. These were a result of the *quantitative distribution of energies within the psychic system* (Munroe 1957), and the essential feature of psychotic conditions was the greater depth of the regression. It is this central concept of regression which plays such an important part in Freud's theory of the neuroses and psychoses. The type of disorder is dependent upon the organism's reaction to conflict by regression. In the case of the psychotic disorders, the regression is more severe, though this distinction between neurosis and psychosis is often blurred, since neurotics may often show breaks with reality. In its simplest form, the Freudian view is that neurosis can be conceived as an intermediate stage along a single dimension, with normality at one end and psychosis at the other. 'Neuroses and psychoses are not separated by a hard and fast line, any more than health and neurosis' (1923, vol XIX, p. 204).

Wexler (1971), however, has suggested that this is representative only of Freud's earlier position (e. g. *Neuropsychoses of Defence* 1894), and that Freud later adopted the view that schizophrenia was to be sharply contrasted with neurosis. In his article, however, Wexler does not make it clear whether he is claiming that Freud rejected the unidimensional model, or simply that he claimed that the disorders were a result of different processes. The latter point is certainly true (see *Neurosis and Psychosis*), but this has little bearing on the unidimensional model.

In an empirical study of 100 schizophrenic, neurotic and normal subjects, Bellak et al. (1973) looked at the adequacy of 'ego function' in these three groups. Scores which were based upon judgements of the person's characteristic level of functioning were presented for reality testing, sense of reality, defensive functioning, autonomous functioning, etc. In all, scores were presented for 11 ego functions, and in each case the psychotics were significantly more disturbed than neurotics, and the neurotics more than normals. The authors examined some of the ways in which their data might be distorted. There was a slight tendency, for instance, for the ego-function ratings to correlate positively with social class, educational level and IQ and negatively with age. The objection might be raised that the concept of ego function is itself sufficiently vague to reflect more about the rater's own notions of psychopathology than about the subject's behaviour. However, this evidence if taken at face value is clearly supportive of the psycho-analytic position. The mean values for the ego function scores are presented in Fig. 2. This illustrates the single dimension and the overlap of the three conditions that is generally assumed by psycho-analysts.

A number of psychiatrists have also taken this unidimensional position, though without the psycho-analytic assumptions about psychosexual regression. Myerson (1936) restated the case that neuroses span the bridge between normal mental states and certain psychotic states, and this unidimensional perspective has prompted most psychiatric interest in the area of depression. It has been suggested that because of the importance of depressive disorders in psychological medicine, any failure to demonstrate two indepen-

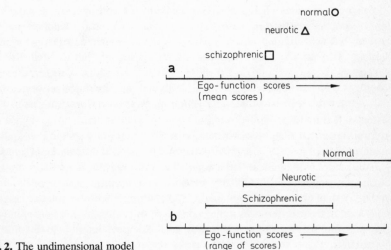

Fig. 2. The undimensional model

dent factors for the depressive conditions would severely limit the value of the separate concepts of neuroticism and psychoticism (Trouton and Maxwell 1956).

In the case of the depressive disorders, most psycho-analysts would accept the unidimensional model. Fenichel (1945) wrote that the difference between neurotic and psychotic depression is one of the depth of narcissistic regression. Mendelson (1974) regards this as a fair summary of the views of both Freud and Rado. This sort of unidimensional point of view has also received considerable support from such influential psychiatrists as Lewis and Mapother in their discussions of neurotic depression. Mapother (1925) denied that there was any fundamental difference between the nature of neurotic and psychotic depressions. Lewis (1934) has also made this point about the neurotic and psychotic types of depression (which he suggests are not to be regarded as synonymous with reactive and endogenous depression). Lewis was impressed by the difficulty of making any qualitative distinctions. The patient who appeared to show reactive depression to a bereavement might have proved to have had a mood change beforehand, and the patient overwhelmed by guilt and self-reproach at one stage could later become angry and hostile. In an analysis of 70 cases admitted to a military hospital, Tredgold (1941) also failed to differentiate two groups of depressives, since many showed typically neurotic and typically psychotic clinical pictures at different stages of their illness.

In a study of over 1000 unselected admissions to the Maudsley Hospital, Kendell (1975) collected 60 different items of information relative to the distinction between neurotic and psychotic depression for each patient and subjected this data to a discriminant function analysis. The distribution of scores was unimodal rather than bimodal, and Kendell concluded that the depressive disorders are best regarded in terms of a single continuum between the neurotic and psychotic states. Kendell acknowledged that the neurotic and endogenous states of depression differ, but like Aubrey Lewis he regarded the majority of cases as falling between the two extremes. When further analysis failed to show any discrete cluster for neurotic depression (Everitt et al. 1971), the authors concluded that psychotic depression is a more firmly based concept than neurotic depression.

After earlier assertions of the validity of the distinction between neurotic and endogenous depressive states (Kiloh and Garside 1965), Kiloh appears to have changed his opinion on this matter. On the basis of factor analytic results, Kiloh et al. (1972) have argued that neurotic depression is a vague concept which 'as a distinct syndrome is an artefact'. It is not clear whether these comments suggest that Kendell, Kiloh and their colleagues are moving towards a position denying the validity of neurotic depression as a disorder altogether. Certainly Kiloh et al. argued that the diagnosis of neurotic depression is often made by excluding endogenous depression and that the disorder is likely to be vague and heterogeneous.

Another study which provided support for the continuity position was made by Garmany (1958) using 525 depressed patients. He found that situational stress factors of various kinds could be identified among 95% of the reactive depression and among 79% of the endogenous cases. Similarly, constitutional predisposing factors could be found among 70% of endogenous depressions and among 55% of the reactive cases. Garmany suggests that these differences are not sufficient to justify any clear differentiation of the two types and that the distinction is really one of degree, that is, between mild and severe depressions.

Table 2. Different approaches to depression

	Categorical model	Dimensional model
One sort of depression	Mapother, Lewis	Freud, Kendall
Two sorts of depression	Kiloh et al.	Eysenck

There are, however, two issues involved in this problem, and much confusion has resulted from a failure to identify them. There is the problem of whether or not neurotic/reactive and psychotic/endogenous depression should be conceptually separated, and of the relative merits of categorical and dimensional frameworks. Four possible positions can be adopted in the dispute, and these are shown in Table 2. The traditional psychiatric position regards neurotic and psychotic depression as two distinct entities (see Kiloh and his colleagues), and it was against this view that Mapother and Lewis first reacted. Freud and Kendell differ from this view in their use of a dimensional framework. The two-dimensional system is best exemplified in the work of Eysenck (1970), who argued that Kendell's unidimensional factor solution is inadequate and severely limited as a framework within which to classify the depressive disorders.

The unimodal hypothesis has also been strongly challenged by Carney et al. (1965), who used similar methods to Kendell and reached a quite different conclusion. The results of their factor analysis show that a bimodal factor accounted for a greater part of the variance than a general factor, and that the various statistical analyses broadly matched the clinical descriptions of neurotic and psychotic depression. Their results could not be accounted for in terms of a single depressive disorder, though the factor loadings suggested that the two disorders did have some features in common. This suggests, therefore, that there are quantitative as well as qualitative differences between the depressive conditions, but that the two dimensions are best regarded as independent of each other.

Burt (1954) described factor analysis as the best statistical device for resolving the problems of classification, and several psychologists have relied heavily upon factor analytic methods in their work. Eysenck and Eysenck (1975) see factor analysis as a necessary, but not a sufficient, method for isolating the main dimensions of personality. The main weakness of this method is its dependence upon correlation, and Eysenck has pointed to the need for personality research to be firmly related to the main body of experimental psychology. Eysenck (1955) firmly rejects the discontinuity model of psychological disorders: neurosis is to be seen as the extreme end of a normal-neurotic continuum.

In order to test the one- and two-dimensional hypotheses about the relationship between neurosis and psychosis, Eysenck (1955) gave four tests (of visual acuity, object recognition, mental speed and visual accommodation) to three groups of normal, neurotic and psychotic subjects. Eysenck argued that these tests had the advantage of being based upon objective rather than interpretative data (their relevance to abnormal psychology is discussed in the paper itself). Using a discriminant function analysis the results supported the view that neurotic and psychotic disorders lie along different and independent dimensions. Loevinger (1955) criticised Eysenck's conclusion that this evidence is contrary to the Freudian unidimensional model on the grounds that the measures chosen have no direct relevance to the particular dimension proposed by Freud.

S. B. G. Eysenck has discussed this issue in the context of 'mixed states', in which it is not clear whether the patient has a neurotic or a psychotic disorder. The clinical textbook definitions tend to focus upon the presence of hallucinations, delusions and cognitive deterioration as evidence of psychosis. Unfortunately, such typical syndromes are rarely encountered in practice. The unidimensional view that neurotic and psychotic disorders differ only in terms of their severity suggests that the difficulty in such cases is due to the patient's presenting 'borderline' symptoms. That is, the severity of the patient's disorder is placed on the continuum between two clear-cut disorders, and therefore includes features of both. As the severity of the disorder increases, it is likely to show the psychotic features more clearly until these have displaced the neurotic symptomatology. If the disorder becomes less severe, the neurotic symptoms will predominate as the patient moves back towards normality. The two-dimensional perspective, on the other hand, accepts the independence of neuroses and psychoses. It is, therefore, possible that the 'mixed-state' cases are simultaneously suffering from both neurotic and psychotic disorders, and that each may vary in severity independently of the other.

In her study (S. B. G. Eysenck 1956) three groups of normal, neurotic and psychotic subjects completed a number of psychological tests. On several of the tests the results of the simple analyses of variance appear to support the unidimensional model; the normals performed best, the psychotics, worst, and the neurotics were in between. On other tests, however, the neurotics were the most disordered group (in terms of their psycho-galvanic response to stressful stimuli, and in the number of abnormal responses to the Maudsley Medical Questionnaire). On the manual dexterity test, on which the psychotics performed worst, Eysenck suggested that the impairment in performance for the two abnormal groups may be a result of different processes. Psychotics may be slow because of their mental retardation, whereas the neurotics may be adversely affected by their anxiety. In the discriminant function analysis, two latent routes were found, each of which were significant beyond the 0.1% level: it was impossible to account for the test responses of the three groups in terms of only one dimension. Eysenck sees these findings as strongly indicative of the independence of neurosis and psychosis.

Eysenck uses a single, general neuroticism factor and locates the various neurotic disorders within a three-dimensional personality framework. Cattell, who also based his system on factor analysis, regards neurosis as a more complex multi-factor concept: anxiety is an important part of neurosis, but it is only one of several dimensions making up the higher-order factor. The Derogatis studies suggest that five basic factors may constitute the core dimensions of neurosis (Derogatis et al. 1970, 1971a, 1971b), and O'Connor (1953) obtained seven factors from an analysis of the symptom clustering of over 300 male neurotic out-patients: again, no general factor of neurosis emerged.

Cattell and Scheier (1961) suggest that Eysenck and the psycho-analysts (an unlikely combination!) both oversimplify neurosis by presenting it as a uni-factor concept. Psycho-analysis accounts for neurosis in terms of regression, and Eysenck through a largely constitutional neuroticism factor. Cattell argues that neither in terms of first-order, nor second-order factors do neurotics differ from normals on only one general factor. To some extent this conflict between single-factor and multi-factor concepts of neurosis reflects differences in the use of factor analytic methods and differences in the type of input data used. It also has much to do with the theoretical persuasions of the investigators.

Cattell has given close consideration to the question of whether neurosis is functionally separable from psychosis. Among the evidence that suggests that the two general types of disorder may usefully be differentiated, Cattell and Scheier (1961) point to the larger hereditary component that seems demonstrable for the psychotic disorders. Also, considering how unreliable specific psychiatric diagnoses can be, there is a relative absence of confusion of the neurotic and psychotic classes of diagnosis.

In a series of studies, Cattell contrasted the questionnaire data (16PF) obtained from 480 clinically judged psychotics and 201 neurotics. The questionnaire profiles of the two groups are different, and when compared with normal subjects, the factors that distinguish neurotics from normal groups are not the same as those which differentiate between psychotics and normals (Cattell and Scheier 1961). Nor did the factors that differentiated between normal and neurotic groups distinguish between normals and psychotics. The bulk of the MMPI research data also points to important differences between neurotic and psychotic groups (Gough 1946; Meehl 1946; Rosen 1962; Silver and Sines 1961), and Cattell, like Eysenck, concluded that the neurotic and psychotic dimensions should be regarded as separate and independent.

Part II

Theories of Neurosis

4. Conditioning Theories of Neurosis

If it is accepted that the modification of the central nervous system through experience is the basis of most, if not all, human and animal behaviour, it should be clear why modern learning theory plays an important role in psychology. Learning and conditioning are pervasive determinants of behaviour, and insofar as the neurotic reactions are also learned reactions, they too are dependent upon the laws of learning (Eysenck 1959). Eysenck places great stress on the importance of experimental studies of learning and conditioning, and of learning theory for an understanding of the neurotic disorders. Joseph Wolpe, another figure whose name is closely associated with the classical conditioning model, has made the same point (Wolpe 1970).

Both Eysenck and Wolpe would accept the following general definition of neurotic symptomatology, that it is *a persisting pattern of learned behaviour which (for some reason) is maladaptive.* Neurotic behaviour fails to achieve its objective and leaves the person dissatisfied and frustrated by his failure. Wolpe tends to be more prescriptive in his definitions by emphasising anxiety, including within his (1970) definition of the neurotic disorders that such behaviour be acquired in anxiety-generating situations; and suggesting that the core of neurotic behaviour lies not in any particular behaviour or motor activity, but in anxiety itself, which is usually the central constituent of neurosis and is *always* present in the causal situations (Wolpe 1958).

Like so many other concepts in abnormal psychology, that of anxiety is evasive; Wolpe defines it as *the responses predominantly of the autonomic nervous system with which the individual characteristically responds to painful or noxious stimuli.* Among its most common manifestations are rapid perspiration, rapid pulse rate, increased blood pressure and a fairly general elevation of muscle tension. A similar specification of the characteristics of neurotic behaviour was made by Eysenck (1975b). Neurotic behaviour is (a) learned and not due to injury or lesions; (b) maladaptive: and (c) involves strong emotions, particularly anxiety. Sidman (1964) has suggested that anxiety is an almost ubiquitous phenomenon and that not all anxiety is neurotic. When faced by a realistic threat, anxiety becomes a normal response. It has been suggested that fear is a more appropriate term to use in this context. Anxiety is seen as neurotic when it appears in the absence of any objective danger. Eysenck and Rachman (1965), however, distinguish between those neurotic reactions such as phobias, anxiety states, obsessional and compulsive disorders, in which anxiety plays a large part, and other disorders which are the result of a failure of conditioning, and in which anxiety plays little part.

4.1 Classical Conditioning

The early classical conditioning model of neurosis proposed by Watson (Watson and Rayner 1920) seems to have equated the neurotic disorder with (Pavlovian) conditioned emotional responses. However, this model in its simplest form has had comparatively little influence, possibly because of the failure of later investigators to replicate Watson's findings (e. g. Bregman 1934), but also because of certain fairly obvious inherent short-comings. Eysenck (1976) proposed an updated version of a conditioning theory of neurosis described as the third conditioning model, of which Watson's was the first, and Mowrer's, the second. But before dealing with the weaknesses of Watson's simple conditioning model and Mowrer's modified version, there are certain issues which can be interpreted in the light of a comparatively straightforward classical conditioning model.

In the case of nocturnal enuresis, which has been regarded as a manifestation of profound underlying emotional disturbances, passive-aggressive feelings towards the parents, or as a substitute form of repressed sexuality, Mowrer's (1938) simple conditioning-deficit model was refreshingly straightforward. In this case there is an apparent failure to connect enlargement of the bladder and the beginning of urination with the appropriate response of waking up and going to the toilet. Mowrer (1976) described how during the late 1930s he became convinced that Pavlovian conditioning could provide an account of the development of nocturnal enuresis and a model for its treatment. The process of conditioning which accounts for the normal waking response is shown in Fig. 3. The conditioning establishes a connection between distention of the bladder and the person waking up and inhibiting the urination. In the enuretic individual there is a failure to wake up and prevent urination. Mowrer's answer to this problem was the by now well-known pad-and-bell apparatus, which enables the establishment of the missing learned connection between distention of the bladder and waking.

More ambitiously, Eysenck (1960b, 1977) has analysed delinquency and antisocial behaviour in similar terms, arguing that conscience may be regarded as a conditioned anxiety response to certain types of situations and actions. The child who behaves in some socially undesirable way, by lying, stealing, being aggressive or whatever, is frequently punished: this leads to pain or fear, with the associated autonomic reactions, and these become associated with the type of situation or type of action which led to the punishment. Similar sequences of events, through the process of stimulus generalisation, establish a conditioned response to a class of antisocial responses, and this generalisation is usually aided by verbal labelling. In the case of the delinquent child, there has been a

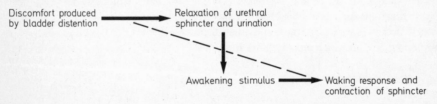

Fig. 3

failure of the conditioning process such that the child has not acquired the internal restraints necessary to prevent him from behaving badly. In fact, Eysenck's explanation of such phenomena is closely linked to a separate theory of individual differences, in which extraverts show weaker conditioned responses than introverted subjects. This is discussed at greater length in Chap. 7.

The reduction of conscience to generalised conditioned avoidance responses has met with considerable resistance, though there are sufficient experimental demonstrations, both with children and animals, to establish that behaviour can be guided in this manner. Solomon et al. (1968), for instance, conducted an experiment with dogs in which the animals were conditioned to avoid an initially preferred food and to choose an initially non-preferred food. The dogs which had been trained with a short delay of punishment quickly learned to confine their eating to the directed food. Delayed punishment produced a less effective conditioned restraint, and the behaviour of the animals was furtive and unreliable. Solomon regarded these experimental procedures as directly comparable to those involved in childhood socialisation, and Mowrer (1950) emphasised that neurotic disorders could best be regarded as examples of under-learning, and both enuresis and the failure to acquire moral restraints were interpreted in this light.

Eysenck and Rachman (1965), however, have also drawn attention to a rather different problem in which the neurotic behaviour may be seen as the result of positive, appetitive conditioning to stimuli contrary to the social, moral or legal requirements of a particular country. Fetishistic behaviour and homosexuality are cited as examples of this sort of behaviour, in which erotic behaviour patterns have been conditioned to particular stimuli, possibly through orgasm, but possibly by other means. This category of 'neurotic' disorders is surrounded by much controversy, since any decision to include such behaviour within the realm of abnormal psychology cannot be divorced from morality and value-judgment. In the case of homosexuality, for instance, the homosexuality itself may have only minor implications for the personality development of the individual. It is the attitudes of others towards this behaviour that are most likely to create the stresses and anxieties which affect personality and social integration. Many adult homosexuals strongly deny that they have any need for psychological help and are insulted by the offer of 'treatment' (Schofield 1965). Siegelman (1978) found that homosexuals scored higher on measures of neuroticism than heterosexual subjects, though this may be related more to feminity (in both sexes) than to sexual preference itself, and Adelman (1977), who gave the MMPI to groups of professionally employed lesbians and heterosexual women, found no evidence of higher levels of neuroticism among the lesbians, though this group did feel more socially alienated than the heterosexual women.

The complexity of the notion of neurosis, incorporating as it does not only individual symptomatology and subjective distress, but also self-perceptions and the social reactions of others, has already been discussed in earlier chapters, and this is not the place to restate these issues. However, there are few areas in abnormal psychology which pose quite so many problems as this of learned preferences (particularly sexual) which also call forth social disapproval. One may or may not choose to regard such behaviour as appropriate material for psychotherapy, though the individual may experience considerable personal distress because of his homosexual, fetishistic, pedophiliac (or whatever) preferences. Although the persistence of such forms of sexual behaviour may lead to socially aversive consequences which may in some cases outweigh their rewarding consequences, one would wish to avoid equating behaviour which receives social disapprobation with neurosis as psychopathology, though Flew (1978) has noted a similar recurrent error in discussions of criminality.

But quite apart from the problem of how one chooses to categorise particular sexual preferences, there is some evidence that classical conditioning procedures can produce positive sexual responses. Rachman and Hodgson (1968) were able to condition a number of male subjects to give a sexual response to previously neutral stimuli (photographs of knee-length boots) in the manner of fetishistic attraction, and Beech et al. (1971) were able to use this sort of classical conditioning paradigm in the successful treatment of a young man with deviant sexual tastes. The simple conditioning model, however, is inadequate here, since in the typical fetishist the individual's sexual desire for, and responses to, the fetishistic object are stronger than to the sexual object itself. Indeed, the fetishists who see a clinician are likely to require the fetishistic object as an indispensable stimulus for the occurrence of any response to the primary sexual object. These aspects of fetishism are not explained by the simple conditioning theory.

There are also problems for a simple conditioning theory in accounting for the more traditional neurotic reactions such as anxiety states, obsessional and compulsive disorders and phobic reactions. In the first place, the limitation of unconditioned stimuli to pain and fear presupposes that neuroses develop as a result of traumatic single trial conditioning or multiple sub-traumatic conditioning. Except in a few exceptional cases, for instance in some war neuroses or in simple phobic reactions, it is comparatively rare to find such 'natural' fear producers at the beginning of a neurosis (Eysenck 1975 b, 1976).

4.2 Conflict and Frustration

Conflict is one factor that has been suggested as a link between exposure to punishment and neurosis, and Dollard and Miller (1950) regarded conflict as the primary cause of the neurotic's unhappiness.

Pavlov (1927) first reported that experimental neuroses could be induced in animals, and classical conditioning theorists have placed considerable weight upon such experimental results. In Pavlov's 'circle and ellipse' experiment, the animal was conditioned to associate the circle with food and the elliptical stimulus with no reward. Having established these conditioned responses, the shape of the ellipse was gradually approximated to that of the circle. When the ratio of the semi-axes of the ellipse reached 9 : 8, the close resemblance of the ellipse to the circle produced a dramatic effect upon the animal's behaviour. The dog, which had previously been a quiet animal, began to squeal and struggle in the apparatus, and when it was taken into the experimental room it would bark violently. Wolpe (1970) referred to this as a state of conflict produced by the strong simultaneous activation of opposite action tendencies – the evocation and inhibition of the alimentary responses. This conflict led to a high level of autonomic arousal which became conditioned to the environmental stimuli of the laboratory. Other investigators were later to use similar methods involving such forms of conflict to produce experimental neuroses. Jacobsen et al. (1935), for instance, obtained experimental neuroses in chimpanzees by presenting discrimination tasks too difficult for the animal, which became angry and emotionally aroused by its errors. There are, of course, many difficulties involved in the attempt to translate these findings into the human neuroses, though the essential issue is not whether the external behaviour is in all respects the same in man and animal, but whether the mechanisms controlling the behaviour are the same or not (Hebb 1947). Wolpe (1952) examined the similarities between the two and argued that experimental and clinical neuroses are parallel phenomena.

The use of the term 'conflict' in these accounts must not be misunderstood; it has no relationship to the psycho-dynamic notion of 'unconscious conflict' between the ego and the id (or super-ego and id), as proposed by Freud. The source of anxiety in this case is quite different. Pavlov, for instance, regarded conflict as the simultaneous elicitation of positive and negative conditioned responses which he related to the physiology of the central nervous system. A more behavioural discussion of the same problem was provided by Neal Miller, whose gradient model of conflict was derived from the work of Hull (1932). Miller (1959) suggested that the nearer the subject is to a goal-object, the stronger is the tendency to approach that object: equally, the tendency to avoid a feared stimulus increases as the subject gets nearer to it. In addition, Miller found it necessary to postulate that the strength of avoidance increases more rapidly with proximity to the goal than does that of approach.

More recently, Miller's proposals have been challenged by Hearst (1969), whose experiments showed that the gradients of approach and avoidance depended upon the specific parameters of the behavioural task. By careful manipulation of the experimental condition, Hearst was able to produce either a steep or a flat approach gradient and either a steep or a flat avoidance gradient. Hearst suggested that there was probably no profound difference in the nature of approach and avoidance behaviour as originally suggested by Miller, and that research might concentrate more profitably upon the particular parameters that flatten or steepen gradients, regardless of approach or avoidance.

This does not, however, lessen the conceptual value of the distinction between approach and avoidance. There are various types of conflict that can be proposed; in their simplest form, these are approach-approach, avoidance-avoidance and approach-avoidance conflict. Teasdale (1974) has suggested that the avoidance-avoidance paradigm can be most profitably applied to the obsessional-compulsive disorders. The obsessional-compulsive patient is seen as being caught in the conflict of whether to perform his rituals or not. If he does, he avoids the feared aversive consequences which might follow non-performance; but the performance itself is hypothesised to lead to other aversive consequences, hence the conflict. Teasdale's analysis, however, assumes that the rituals are avoidance responses which save the person from aversive consequences, which may be probable, but leaves unexplained the fact that obsessionals may sometimes stop performing their rituals or even deliberately engage in acts of contamination (Beech and Perigault 1974).

Also, Teasdale suggests that the oscillation between two alternative responses that is characteristic of laboratory avoidance-avoidance conflict, has been described in clinical accounts of the behaviour of obsessional-compulsive patients who were in doubt as to whether or not to perform their rituals (e. g. Mather 1970). It is not clear, however, why the patient should sometimes perform the ritual and sometimes avoid doing so. The suggestion that the ritual is performed because the overall aversiveness of the consequences of performance of the ritual is less than that following non-performance (Teasdale 1974) is unhelpful because it falls so quickly into tautology.

Others have suggested that approach-avoidance conflict may provide a more useful model for the analysis of the neurotic disorders (e. g. Maher 1966). The approach-avoidance conflict is a form of passive avoidance learning, in which the animal is simultaneously attracted to and repelled by the same stimulus. Miller asserted that conflict generates drive, and being part of the Hullian tradition, maintained Hull's uni-process view of learning, looking to drive reduction as the source of reinforcement.

Gray (1971) applied Miller's analysis to sexual deviations, suggesting that such phenomena as voyeurism and fetishism could be seen as examples of the conflict between heterosexual approach tendencies and avoidance tendencies, and that such psychosomatic disorders as stomach ulcers can be caused by conflict and helplessness. Gray also referred to the interesting series of studies discussed by Azrin and Holz (1966). In one of their experiments (Holz and Azrin 1961), these authors punished the responses of the subject animal during the period of reinforcement. The result of this procedure was to reverse completely the usual effects of punishment – the rate of responding increased in the presence of punishment and decreased in its absence. Punishment when followed by reward can acquire secondary reinforcing properties. This finding is extremely interesting and may well have a certain bearing upon such human disorders as masochism, in which a person becomes aroused by things which most of us would regard as painful or humiliating. Gray (1971) has also pointed to the way in which masochism may be explained in terms of the pairing of reward and punishment such that punishment becomes a sign of reward.

Dollard and Miller (1950) presented one of the more explicit early statements of the effects of conflict upon neurosis. In the case of approach-avoidance conflict, Dollard and Miller saw this as the sort of conflict which usually occurred between the responses of trying to think about or remember something and the response of repression; equally it could be seen as the sort of conflict which occurred when the neurotic is prevented by his inhibitions from achieving his goal. These authors also regard the neurotic patient as a specially selected case with unusually strong avoidance tendencies. Any attempts to increase the patient's motivation to achieve his thwarted goals in life are likely only to increase the level of conflict and therefore his misery, and Dollard and Miller suggested that the therapist should begin his work by reducing the fears which cause the avoidance. Most behaviour therapists would probably accept that conflict may play an important role in the development of experimental and clinical neuroses through its aversive properties (Chesser 1976). It is not, however, accepted as a necessary cause of anxiety neuroses, and Wolpe (1958) has argued that traumatic conditioning is a more likely sufficient cause of such neurotic reactions.

Amsel (1962) assigned a similar function to frustration as a source of drive. Hull's theory failed to acknowledge that the omission of a reward constituted any special sort of event for the subject, and Gleitman et al. (1954) traced some of the difficulties which follow from this. Working within a neo-Hullian framework, Amsel described frustrative non-reward as having many of the properties of punishment, and operating in many respects like fear. Indeed, he suggested that the avoidance of non-reward was a more powerful factor in discrimination learning than approach to reward.

Gray (1971) has taken a similar position, arguing that the omission of an expected reward has effects which are very similar to, and may even be identical with, the effects of punishment. In both its functional and physiological effects, frustration (in this sense) can be equated with fear. It is impossible to demonstrate the aversive qualities of non-reward directly, since the termination of non-reward is simply the attainment of reward, but it can be shown that stimuli which have been associated with frustrative non-reward are aversive (Adelman and Maatsch 1956). It is also possible to substitute direct physical punishment for frustrative non-reward and obtain very similar results (Brown and Wagner 1964).

Early accounts of conditioned fear responses emphasised physical pain or fear as the UCR in the conditioning process (cf. Watson). Eysenck (1975b) has argued that this is too restrictive and invoked the notion of frustrative non-reward as a much more likely variable. Actual physical pain and fear are not often easy to find when one tries to determine the characteristics of the situations from which the neurotic reaction developed, though they may be found in the extreme circumstances leading to war neuroses. It is also possible that some simple phobias may be associated with such factors. But with these exceptions, traumatic single trial conditioning, or multiple, sub-traumatic conditioning, with pain or fear as the UCR, cannot provide a satisfactory explanation for the development of most neurotic disorders. Frustrative non-reward has greater plausibility as a UCR in this context.

The use of this concept of frustrative non-reward, however, introduces a cognitive element into the discussion. The absence of reward cannot have specific aversive properties unless the organism *expects* to be rewarded. Eysenck (1979) denied that this makes any fundamental difference to the non-cognitive status of the conditioning theory, on the grounds that cognition can itself be explained in terms of the principles of conditioning. This is hotly disputed by the cognitive theorists (see Chap. 5).

4.3 Two-Stage Theory

One of the greatest obstacles for learning theory in attempting to explain how neuroses develop is the phenomenon of extinction. Unreinforced conditioned reactions extinguish rapidly, yet neurotic reactions appear to contradict this fundamental principle of learning theory. Mowrer (1950) provided one of the clearer statements of this 'neurotic paradox':

> Common sense holds that a normal, sensible man, or even a beast to the limits of his intelligence, will weigh and balance the consequences of his acts: if the net effect is favourable, the action producing it will be perpetuated; and if the net effect is unfavourable, the action producing it will be inhibited, abandoned. In neurosis, however, one sees actions which have predominantly unfavourable consequences; yet they persist over a period of months, years, or a lifetime.

It is because neurotic behaviour runs contrary to the predictions of Thorndike's law of effect and Skinner's principles of reinforcement that a special theory is required.

Mowrer and Ullman (1945) tackled this neurotic paradox of behaviour which persisted, despite the fact that it was more punished than rewarded, and suggested that Hull's (1932, 1943) notion of gradients of reinforcement could be used here. If a response is followed by two consequences, one of which is rewarding and the other punishing, this may lead to persistent non-integrative behaviour. If a weak reward is received before a strong punishment, behaviour may persist despite the greater punishment: equally, if the reward occurs later, behaviour may be inhibited despite its being more rewarding than punishing. In Mowrer's view, neurotic behaviour is best seen as a learning deficit rather than as a case of overlearning, and an explanation of neurosis should deal with the problem of why the neurotic fails to learn, and not with why he fails to unlearn. Like the ostrich, the neurotic is seen as dealing directly with his anxiety by avoiding exposing himself to reality, or at least by delaying the consequences of his actions in the real world.

Mowrer's two-stage theory of neurosis proposed that a neutral stimulus comes to elicit anxiety as a result of classical conditioning. This learning is then protected from extinction by the second stage, in which an instrumental avoidance response leads to anxiety reduction and sets up a conditioned avoidance reaction to the CS. The remarkable persistence of the neurotic behaviour can therefore be accounted for in terms of the *immediate* anxiety reduction consequences of the avoidance, against the *delayed* negative effects of such behaviour. In psychiatric terms, this behaviour can be interpreted as the avoidance of 'reality testing' (Eysenck 1976).

Strictly speaking, Miller's theory was a one-stage theory rather than a two-stage theory like that of Mowrer. Miller regarded learning very much in Hullian terms, as a process of drive reduction, and thought that the original fear response was itself learned on the basis of *fear reduction*. Gray (1975) has reviewed the evidence in support of this position and concluded that it is incompatible with the weight of empirical evidence. What both theorists agree upon is that the person or animal in an active avoidance situation does not learn to avoid the punishment but to terminate the stimuli which are followed by punishment. Both, therefore, rely heavily upon the motivating properties of anxiety/fear reduction; (Miller [1948] showed that conditioned fear stimuli were indeed aversive). The fear and anxiety are seen to motivate and reinforce behaviour that avoids or prevents the recurrence of the aversive unconditioned stimulus (Mowrer 1939).

The unusual circumstances of warfare which produced 'war neuroses' have been cited by several authors in support of their argument. Dollard and Miller (1950) referred to the case of a pilot who developed a phobic fear of aeroplanes as a result of his traumatic experiences in combat. The fear resulting from the initial trauma of combat became associated with the aeroplane and generalised to other aeroplanes: this fear motivated his avoidance, which in turn was reinforced by the reduction in the strength of his fear. In the case of the war neuroses, the trauma of combat was usually counteracted by a process of enforced extinction in the front line. By removing the person to a base hospital, the conditioned fear response would be protected from extinction in the same way that the avoidance response protects the first stage of learning. As early as 1926, and contrary to the predominantly psycho-dynamic orientation of military psychiatry at that time, Fenton wrote that 'shell-shock' could be understood in terms of the laws of habit formation.

Among the more common neurotic disorders, Mowrer (1969) has discussed the psycho-neurotic defences (for example, deception and denial) as punishment-avoidance strategies. In particular, he examined the ways in which the subject can perform a forbidden act without getting punished or refrain from performing a required response and still avoid punishment. Under these circumstances, the person is likely to experience conflict due to the opposing requirements of the situation. Lying and deceit are ways of reducing the original conflict, though they entail the problems of a further conflict between the guilt resulting from the deceit and the fear of punishment which would occur if the deception were admitted. In passive avoidance situations, Mowrer uses the term 'guilt' to refer to the fear experienced between the performance of the forbidden act and the occurrence of punishment. This distinguishes it from temptation fear. It is not clear if guilt is a relevant feature of active avoidance, since this can be explained quite satisfactorily by the simpler concept of 'fear'.

Two features of neurosis which require explanation are the occurrence of spontaneous recovery in some cases and the massive resistance to extinction in others. Eysenck and Rachman (1965) used a two-stage theory (though they refer to it as a three-stage theory) to explain both. Spontaneous recovery, which they describe as the most obvious, most impressive and least frequently acknowledged aspect of neurotic disorders, is explained as being due to classical conditioning processes only. That is, the first stage of conditioning establishes a learned fear through the association of a neutral CS with the fear-producing UCS, and the CS alone subsequently elicits the original maladaptive emotional response. However, the conditioned autonomic responses extinguish as the person encounters further instances in which the CS presentation is not reinforced. Denker (1946) looked at 500 severe cases of neurosis and found that 70% recovered within 2 years without any form of psychotherapy. After 5 years, over 90% had recovered. To this extent, the classical conditioning account can explain why a substantial majority of neurotics show spontaneous recovery. In order to explain why some cases of neurosis are apparently so resistant to extinction, Eysenck and Rachman (1965) found it necessary to utilise the second stage of instrumental learning. The active avoidance response protects the original learned fear from extinction and is itself reinforced through anxiety reduction.

Dollard and Miller (1950) suggested that compulsive behaviour and hysterical disorders could also be explained by the two-stage theory, and Eysenck and Rachman (1965) argued that all the dysthymic neuroses (anxiety states, phobias, obsessional and compulsive disorders etc.) could be explained in this way. More recently, however, both Eysenck (1968, 1975b, 1976) and Rachman (1976) have recognised the deficiencies of this sort of account and have proposed a number of revisions and extensions.

Among the deficiencies of this theory was its inability to explain the extreme persistence of active avoidance behaviour. Solomon and Wynne (1953) used an adaptation of the Miller-Mowrer shuttle-box to investigate traumatic avoidance learning. Their dogs were trained to avoid an electric shock by responding to a signal preceding the shock. During the escape phase of learning, the animals received shocks, and the latency of the escape response (jumping to the other side of the shuttle-box) gradually decreased. After the onset of the successful avoidance response the latencies continued to decrease, although the animal was no longer being exposed to the noxious UCS. Solomon and Wynne (1954) also described how a few intense shocks during the acquisition of avoidance could lead to hundreds of successful avoidance responses which occurred with fewer and fewer overt signs of anxiety. But according to an unmodified two-stage theory, as the fear of the warning signal declines (this is described by Solomon and Wynne 1953) the avoidance response should also decline, and in the absence of further reconditioning the successful avoidance response should extinguish. Solomon and Wynne dealt with these difficulties by introducing the principle of 'anxiety conservation', which referred to a complex interrelationship between the strength of the anxiety reactions and the instrumental avoidance responses. In those cases where the subject is exposed to a particularly strong UCS which produces intense anxiety, Solomon and Wynne also suggested that the classical conditioning of the emotional response may be partially irreversible.

Several authors have stressed the relative independence of fear and avoidance (e. g. Gray 1971, 1975; Rachman and Hodgson 1974), and Gray has used the notion of 'safety signals' to explain the persistence of active avoidance behaviour. In this way, the fear established in the initial stage could extinguish and still leave the avoidance behaviour intact. The safety signals possess reinforcing properties established by classical conditioning (Rescorla 1969) and are as effective as warning signals in maintaining active avoidance (Bolles 1970; Bolles and Grossen 1969). In this way, successful avoidance behaviour could be ascribed to reinforcement provided by the accompanying safety signals even when there was no conditioned stimulus for the organism to terminate. Nonetheless, this modification of the Mowrer two-stage theory is not entirely satisfactory, since it is difficult to see how avoidance behaviour could ever spontaneously extinguish under such conditions.[1]

4.4 Incubation

Wolpe (1958) drew attention to a number of experimental findings that present other difficulties for any learning theory. These show that in many cases not only does the unreinforced CS fail to extinguish, but it actually produces more and more anxiety (the conditioned response) with each presentation of the CS. Eysenck (1976) also discussed this phenomenon, which even more than the failure of extinction seems to constitute the central paradox of the neuroses. Eysenck (1975b, 1976) has argued that the law of extinction as originally stated is in need of major revision, and has suggested that the presentation of an unreinforced CS (symbolised as $\overline{CS}$) which has been associated with a pain, fear or anxiety-producing UCS may have two separate and contradictory effects. The $\overline{CS}$ may produce (a) extinction of the CR and (b) enhancement of the CR.

The specific outcome in any case will depend upon the strength of the UCR, the duration of the CS and the emotionality of the individual. Grant (1964) distinguished between *Pavlovian A conditioning,* which is exemplified by Pavlov's bell-salivation experiments, and *Pavlovian B conditioning.* This distinction has not perhaps received the attention that it deserves, since its implications are of particular importance for a conditioning theory of neurosis. Eysenck (1979) has argued that neurosis may only be understood in terms of Pavlovian B conditioning.

This can be illustrated by an experiment in which the experimental animal is given repeated injections of morphine which lead to nausea, increased salivation and vomiting. After repeated injections the animal begins to show nausea, vomiting etc. when approached by the experimenter (Pavlov 1927). In Pavlovian B conditioning the UCS is not contingent upon the subject's behaviour, is less dependent for its effect upon the subject's motivational state, and the CS acts as a partial substitute for the UCS. In addition the UCS elicits the complete UCR.

Eysenck (1968) suggested that anxiety has certain peculiar properties which distinguish it from other types of conditioned responses (with the possible exception of sexual CRs). Anxiety has secondary drive properties and is also a source of secondary reinforcement (the primary drive involved acting through pain or frustrative non-reward). 'Neutral stimuli associated with pain give rise to anxiety-fear responses ... and the proprioceptive consequences of these learned responses produce the drive stimuli (^{S}D) that serve the secondary drive' (Eysenck 1975b). The conditioned pain reaction resembles the unconditioned pain reaction in that both have the drive-producing and reinforcing

---

1 For the determined reader who wishes to immerse himself in the intricacies of two-stage theories of avoidance learning, Gray's (1975) discussion can be recommended.

properties of primary drives. In Eysenck's account it is essential to distinguish between CRs that do have drive properties and those that do not. Conditioned stimuli which do not produce drives are subject to the classical law of extinction. Those CSs that do produce drives lead to an enhancement or *incubation* of the CR. This is because when anxiety (or another response with drive properties) is being conditioned, it is not true to say that the CS is not being reinforced in the absence of the UCS. After conditioning, the CS itself produces fear/anxiety.

The CS and $\overline{CS}$ both come to signal danger and punishment. Eysenck terms these consequences NRs – for nocive or noxious responses, to distinguish them from UCRs and CRs. Each NR which follows a CS represents a reinforcement and increases the habit strength associating stimulus and response. This incubation effect in the absence of the UCS and UCR is shown in Fig. 4. Although it may be a much weaker form of reinforcement than that accompanying the UCS, the presence of the NR would theoretically lead to incubation. The conditioning has in this case established a positive feedback cycle in which the CR (NR) provides reinforcement for the CS. More accurately one might say that it is not the CR itself, but the response-produced stimuli, the fear/anxiety, that acts as reinforcer (Eysenck 1979). An electric shock is followed by pain; the $\overline{CS}$ is followed by fear. Shock + CS is followed by fear and pain (NR). This combined NR is more unpleasant than either on its own and therefore has greater reinforcing properties. The $\overline{CS}$ is followed by fear, which although less reinforcing than pain and fear, may still be sufficiently reinforcing to offset the extinction and lead to an incubation effect.

As a clinical illustration of this process, Eysenck (1975) presents two cases – one of insomnia and one of sexual impotence. In the case of a man who finds himself impotent on one occasion due to drink, fatigue or illness, the CSs associated with this occasion produce anxiety as a CR. On the next occasion, these CRs (or NRs) follow the $\overline{CS}$ and

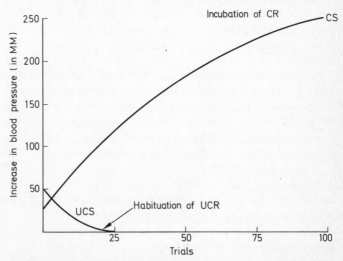

Fig. 4. The incubation effect. The increase in blood pressure as a function of repeated exposure to the UCS (habituation) or to the CS-only. Presentation of the CS alone led to an incubation of the CR (Eysenck 1975b). I am grateful to Professor Eysenck for allowing me to use this illustration

cause reciprocal inhibition of the sexual responses. This failure increases the strength of the anxiety CRs and sets up the conditions for the positive feedback to establish the impotence without any repetition of the original CS-UCS presentation.

As well as its value in explaining features of the dysthymic neuroses, the incubation effect can also be applied to neurotic disorders of the second kind. In fetishism, for instance, the sexual responses to the fetishistic object are often stronger than the primary sexual object. A simple conditioning theory cannot account for this. However, sexual responses, like anxiety, possess drive properties, and the incubation paradigm may be used to explain the development of fetishistic behaviour in the absence of a CS-UCS pairing.

Eysenck (1976) has also pointed out that the duration of CS-only exposure is an important factor, and that short periods of exposure to the CS on its own are likely to produce incubation, whereas long periods of exposure to the CS-only produce extinction. This has clear implications for response-prevention or 'flooding' therapies, since the use of short CS exposures may have an adverse effect. In one instance, a phobic patient who had been exposed to a number of brief (2-min) sessions of CS-only presentations of her phobic stimuli reported that her fear increased during treatment (Rachman 1966).

4.5 The Stimulus

We have largely taken the concept of the 'stimulus' for granted, and few learning theorists have examined the problems associated with this notion. One of the first difficulties with the conditioned stimulus is that in real life the CS is very rarely comparable to the single stimuli which are presented in the usual laboratory experiments; instead, it is much more likely to consist of a variety of interrelated events and objects. In the laboratory the subject is usually exposed to a single clear-cut stimulus which is highly salient because of the controlled conditions, but in real life, classical conditioning theory cannot specify which aspect or aspects of the environment will take on the role of the CS. Early conditioning theory seems to have taken for granted that all potential stimuli were equally associable, but Seligman (1970) has challenged this assumption (as is discussed later in this chapter).

Eysenck (1975b) acknowledged that single, specific conditioned stimuli are rarely found in real-life conditioning, that single-trial traumatic conditioning is exceptional, and that even multiple sub-traumatic conditioning with a single CS is not often observed in the genesis of human neuroses. Eysenck goes on to state that there is no reason why this should invalidate a conditioning theory of neurosis, though the problem clearly becomes far more complex and difficult when there is a multiplicity of conditioned stimuli.

In those cases of neurosis which are characterised by 'free-floating anxiety', it has sometimes been suggested that the conditioning theory is inadequate because of the absence of a specified conditioned stimulus. Wolpe (1967a), however, has argued that anxiety responses can be conditioned to more or less omnipresent properties of the environment which cause the person to become persistently restless and anxious, and suggests that such amorphous features as light, light and shade contrasts, spatiality and even the passage of time can function as conditioned stimuli in classical conditioning. Under such conditions, the patient appears to show a generalised agoraphobia or 'free-floating anxiety', when in fact they are still responding to a CS. Wolpe regards the term 'free-floating anxiety' as a misnomer and has offered 'pervasive anxiety' as a more appropriate description. Wolpe views neurotic behaviour as directed by external stimulation and supports his suggestion that anxiety has specific stimulus sources even in cases of pervasive anxiety disorders by citing clinical evidence.

This sort of analysis of the more generalised neurotic disorders in terms of specific, external conditioned stimuli by Wolpe is interesting, but in danger of becoming tautologous. It is not clear how one could ever provide an example of an anxiety-based neurotic disorder that was not controlled by specific conditioned stimuli if Wolpe is prepared to allow this role to such vague notions as spatiality or the passage of time. The passage of time is, in any case, a highly abstract concept which cannot be said to exist in any real sense except in cognitive terms.

Classical conditioning theory has always been somewhat ambiguous about the role of cognitive factors in determining behaviour. One might infer from the work of S-R theorists that external stimuli have a *direct* impact upon the organism, and that cognitive factors are unimportant. Hearst (1969) stated that, 'the delivery of noxious stimuli to an organism may affect not only the future probability of various responses by the subject, but also the extent to which different stimuli in the external environment control the subject's behaviour.' Conditioning and cognitive theorists have usually resisted explanations couched in terms of the other's concepts and theories, though there have been attempts to reconcile the two in recent years (e. g. Seligman and Johnston 1973).

4.6 Preparedness

A further modification to the simple classical conditioning account has been proposed by Rachman and Seligman (1976) and Eysenck (1976). This involved the concept of *preparedness*.

In a review of the data from traditional learning paradigms, Seligman (1970) showed that the assumption of equivalence – that all events are equally associable and obey common laws – made by general process learning theory is incorrect. In classical conditioning, it is not true that any CS and UCS can be associated with equal facility, nor that the laws governing the rates of acquisition, extinction, spontaneous recovery, etc. are the same for all CSs and UCSs. Nor, in instrumental conditioning, is it the case that the choice of response and reinforcer is a matter of relative indifference. The organism appears to show a preparedness to associate certain stimuli with relative ease, whereas others may be associated only with the greatest difficulty (contra-preparedness).

In one experiment (Garcia and Koelling 1966), rats were exposed to X-rays whenever they drank saccharin-flavoured water. At the same time, they were also exposed to flashing lights and to a noise. The X-irradiation makes the rats sick after a delay of about an hour. When the rats were retested, they had acquired an aversion to the taste of saccharin, but not to the visual and auditory stimuli to which they were also exposed during the experimental sessions. There is a host of experiments which show that rats will readily learn certain responses, such as bar-pressing for food and running to avoid shock, but it is difficult to train rats to press bars to avoid shock (D'Amato and Schiff 1964). Seligman (1970) pointed out the biological utility of the taste-nausea preparedness, and the same can also be said of the preparedness of certain avoidance or appetitive responses. As in other areas (e. g. Maturana et al. 1960; Gossop, 1974), the animal seems prepared to behave most appropriately to stimuli which have clear biological and evolutionary significance for it.

Seligman (1971) has applied this sort of analysis to phobias and pointed out that in general, phobias comprise a relatively limited set of objects. Agoraphobia, fear of certain animals and insects, fear of heights and fear of the dark are common. Fears associated with electricity, hammers or cars are extremely rare, although they are just as likely to be linked with traumatic events. Seligman argued that phobias are highly prepared to be learnt by humans and resistant to extinction: they are instances of prepared conditioning. All stimuli are not equally likely to be transformed into fear signals (Rachman and Seligman 1976), and the preparedness of stimuli is related to their biological significance. Among the clinical implications of this, it has been suggested that *unprepared phobias* are likely to be highly intractable to behaviour therapy, whereas behaviour therapy may be the treatment of choice for prepared phobias (Rachman and Seligman 1976).

4.7 Therapeutic Implications of Conditioning Theory

It will become apparent as the various accounts of neurosis are presented in this book, that different theories have different areas of strength and weakness. Conditioning theory is particularly strong in explaining specific anxiety-linked neurotic symptoms (e. g. phobias and obsessions) and rather weak in dealing with more generalised disorders such as depression.

One therapeutic principle that underlies much of behaviour therapy is that of counter-conditioning, in which the acquisition and strengthening of a new response incompatible with the previous response leads to the elimination of the earlier response (Meyer and Chesser 1970). It has been suggested that anxiety can be directly deconditioned by associating it with an incompatible response, and Wolpe has emphasised the importance of *reciprocal inhibition* in this context. *If a response which inhibits anxiety can be made to occur in the presence of anxiety-evoking stimuli, it will weaken the connection between those stimuli and the anxiety* (Wolpe 1958, 1970). It has even been suggested that despite the theoretical persuasion of the therapist, effective psychotherapy is nearly always based upon reciprocal inhibition of neurotic anxiety responses (Wolpe 1960, 1967b).

Watson and Rayner (1920) suggested that Albert could have been treated by attempts to 'recondition' him in this way, using simultaneous pairings of the fear-producing CS and stimulation of the erogenous zones. Mary Cover-Jones (1924) first demonstrated that neurotic fears in children could be eliminated by pairing a feared CS with pleasant stimuli, and the behaviour therapy literature is now full of accounts confirming and extending the values of treatments based on this procedure. One of the best known treatments is systematic desensitisation based upon relaxation.[2]

Intense muscle relaxation effects are antagonistic to the autonomic arousal associated with anxiety. By presenting a graduated hierarchy of anxiety-provoking stimuli paired with relaxation, the anxiety responses become inhibited. Lazarus and Rachman (1960) suggested that this procedure should be most readily applicable to disorders involving neurotic reactions to concrete and definable stimuli, and in which specific rather than

---

2 The reader is referred to Wolpe (1958) and Wolpe et al. (1973) for a full description of the precise procedures involved in systematic desensitisation.

free-floating anxiety is present. In Wolpe's (1970) view, however, neurotic responses are stimulus-specific even in the case of 'free-floating anxiety' in which anxiety responses have been conditioned to 'more or less omnipresent properties of the environment' such as light, noise or the passage of time (Wolpe 1967a). The term 'pervasive anxiety' is suggested as a better alternative, since in Wolpe's view there is no clear distinction between specific anxiety-provoking stimuli and stimuli to pervasive anxiety. It is, however, generally accepted that patients with multiple fears and extensive social and emotional difficulties are not as good candidates for systematic desensitisation (Wolpe et al. 1973).

In his review of the 75 outcome studies of systematic desensitisation published prior to 1968, Paul (1966) found that the results clearly showed its effectiveness as a treatment for a range of anxiety-based neurotic disorders (including specific phobias as well as agoraphobia, claustrophobia, frigidity and impotence). There are, however, problems in explaining the effects of desensitisation. Benjamin et al. (1972) found that relaxation was a redundant component in the total procedure, and Yates (1975) suggested that every one of the specific components of systematic desensitisation could be removed without leading to therapeutic failure: like the Cheshire cat, desensitisation is left with only its smile. Although Wolpe has emphasised the role of reciprocal inhibition in desensitisation, the effects may equally be explained in terms of counter-conditioning, extinction or habituation. For this reason, although it appears that desensitisation is effective as a treatment for certain neurotic disorders, the critical factors have not been identified, and the theoretical explanations of the effects are conflicting.

It has been suggested, for instance, that exposure to the anxiety-provoking stimuli may be of more importance than relaxation (Marks 1974). Flooding, in which the patient is exposed to intense imaginary or real-life, anxiety-provoking stimuli, is, in terms of stimulus intensity, at the opposite extreme to desensitisation; yet Boulougouris et al. (1971) found that in the treatment of phobic patients, flooding (in fantasy) was superior to desensitisation on clinical and physiological measures, though both treatments led to improvement. Marks et al. (1975) treated 20 patients with chronic obsessive-compulsive rituals by in-vivo exposure with self-imposed response prevention, and they found a significant improvement in compulsive behaviour after 3 weeks, which was maintained at follow-up. Other studies by Rachman et al. (1971) and Hodgson et al. (1972) also suggested that obsessional neuroses improved significantly more with exposure than with relaxation treatments, and flooding may be a more appropriate treatment for agoraphobia than desensitisation. Habituation was suggested as a possible critical feature of the flooding, modelling and relaxation treatments (Rachman et al. 1971), since the patients were prevented from *avoiding exposure* to the anxiety-provoking stimuli. Similarly, response-prevention techniques have been found to be effective with obsessional-compulsive disorders (Meyer and Levy 1970; Levy and Meyer 1971). In this case, the patient is again deliberately exposed to the anxiety-provoking stimuli and the process of extinction is encouraged by the therapist preventing the compulsive thoughts or rituals.

Aversion therapy is one of the best-known, and most controversial, forms of behaviour therapy. It has been used mainly in the treatment of approach responses which cause the patient distress (and which are frequently also the subject of social disapproval). Among these disorders are alcoholism, drug addiction and various sexual disorders such as fetishism, transvestism, voyeurism and, more controversially, homosexuality (e. g. Marks and Gelder 1967; Hallam et al. 1972). In theory, the treatment works by the association of a conditioned aversion with the undesired habit either by presenting a noxious stimulus when the act is performed, or by pairing a noxious stimulus with the stimuli that elicit the behaviour. Again, this eliminates the undesirable behaviour by establishing an incompatible response.

The two sorts of aversive stimulation that have been used in almost all studies are electric shock and various chemical agents. The use of drugs has a number of drawbacks associated with it. The drugs may have a delayed and unpredictable effect, and emetic drugs are obviously messy and unpleasant for the therapist and nursing staff as well as for the patient, and Rachman (1965) has advocated the use of electrical methods. This enables a more precise control of the timing, intensity and duration of the stimulus, and allows the use of partial reinforcement schedules.

Although some interpretations of aversion therapy have relied upon anticipatory avoidance conditioning as the effective underlying principle (Feldman and MacCulloch 1971), there are good reasons to suppose that classical conditioning might be the critical factor (Rachman and Teasdale 1969). Certainly chemical forms of aversion therapy may be explained quite satisfactorily in terms of classical conditioning. In this case, the repeated association between particular stimuli and the UCR of nausea provoked by an emetic drug establishes a conditioned nauseous reaction to the undesirable activity. However, there are considerable difficulties involved in explaining electrical aversion therapy in this way.

According to classical conditioning theory, the pairing of CS with shock should lead to the CS producing a conditioned response of pain/anxiety. In fact, there is comparatively little evidence to support this interpretation. Although Hallam and Rachman (1972) found changes in cardiac responsiveness to sexually deviant stimuli after aversion therapy, other studies found little alteration in physiological function: nor were patients typically found to report feelings of subjective anxiety. Some patients described feelings of indifference to the CS after treatment (Marks and Gelder 1967), and others experienced repulsion rather than anxiety (Hallam et al. 1972). Aversion therapy, like other behaviour therapies, appears to work fairly well; it compares favourably with other treatments for the same disorders, for instance sexual deviations (c. f. Feldman 1966). But the mechanisms by which this and the other behaviour therapies achieve their effect are still not completely understood.

5. Social and Cognitive Theories

In his analysis of the dynamics of scientific investigation, Kuhn (1962) described how science is guided by paradigms. A paradigm has a guidance function, providing an intellectual framework which determines the scientist's views about his subject matter. In psychology, the paradigm or framework within which one operates influences which aspects of human functioning are studied most thoroughly and which are neglected. Psychologists who choose to exclude the capacity for self-direction from their view of human nature will tend to restrict their research focus to external sources of stimulation and control. But although such external influences do have a powerful effect upon human behaviour, it has been argued that the limitation of research to external influences leads to an incomplete and deformed psychological theory (Bandura 1977).

5.1 Dissatisfaction with Conditioning Theories

In recent years there has been a noticeable upsurge of interest in social and cognitive explanations of human behaviour. Kanfer and Phillips (1970) regard this as a reflection of several factors, including an increasing dissatisfaction with learning theories based upon the S-R conditioning model. The human capacity for speech and thought, for instance, is said to have effects upon behaviour which by-pass simple conditioning, and S-R theories have been particularly criticised for their inability to explain the acquisition of novel responses, language, thought and social development.

Pavlov provided the first conditioning interpretation of verbal behaviour, using the concept of a second signalling system which bridged the gap between perceptual and symbolic stimuli, and more recently, others have maintained this view of speech as a set of conditioned responses acquired by the child as a result of his social relationships (Luria 1961). By means of speech and thought, the child enlarges his experience and acquires new modes of behaviour and new ways of actively organising his mental activities; a vital feature of speech (and thought) is that it enables man to go beyond the bounds of his physical capacities. But despite the efforts of Luria and others (e. g. Osgood 1953; Berlyne 1954) to analyse speech, thought and knowledge in S-R terms, the cognitive and social theorists have usually rejected this approach. There are, for instance, many problems involved in a linguistic analysis which uses words as its basic units, since communication is typically based upon sentences rather than isolated word-units, and the meaning of a sentence is not the same as that of the summated meanings of the component words.

There is further dissatisfaction with the lack of any clear and universally accepted definition of such central concepts as stimulus and response, and this creates an area of confusion in the arguments between S-R theories and cognitive theories. Wolpe's (1967) suggestion that abstractions such as 'the passage of time' can function as stimuli is difficult to reconcile with the traditional behavioural emphasis upon external and observable stimuli, responses and reinforcement contingencies. The use of such terms to refer to vague and abstract features of the naturalistic setting outside the laboratory often presents considerable semantic difficulties, and Mahoney et al. (1974) argue that the terminology of conditioning is often used metaphorically in these cases. In Wolpe's attempt to explain pervasive anxiety by reference to the passage of time as a CS, it is easier to accept the cognitive interpretation that the human organism responds primarily to cognitive representations of its environment rather than to the environment itself (Mahoney 1977).

Traditionally, conditioning theorists have suggested that conditioning is an automatic and unconscious process (Thorndike 1932; Dollard and Miller 1950; Wolpe 1978). Brewer (1974) has strongly challenged this view and argued that conditioning (in human subjects) is the result of higher mental processes and not vice versa. Similarly, Bandura (1969, 1974) suggested that in the classical conditioning paradigm the CS comes to produce emotional responses not because it has been invested with emotional properties, but because it elicits emotionally arousing thoughts. Conditioned reactions are largely self-activated on the basis of learnt expectations rather than automatically evoked. The emotional response is cognitively mediated rather than an automatic response to the CS, and from this viewpoint the performance of responses that have been seen to be punished in others can produce anticipatory self-arousal without requiring any emotional response to have been conditioned initially to the CS.

Brewer (1974) asserted that the events in conditioning are a result of the subject's becoming aware of the CS-UCS relationship (in classical conditioning) or of the reinforcement contingency in operant conditioning. Recent investigations have confirmed the early findings of Cook and Harris (1937) that instructions alone are sufficient to elicit and to extinguish the galvanic skin response. Katz et al. (1971) found that simply informing their subjects of the CS-UCS relationship established a conditioned response just as efficiently as actual exposure to CS-UCS parings. Subjects also showed extinction of GSRs within two trials after being told that no further shocks would occur, and the authors regard these results as indicative of cognitive mediation processes.

Conditioning theory and cognitive theory also make opposed predictions about the outcome of experiments in which the subject is exposed to a standard conditioning procedure, but is deceived as to the nature of the CS-UCS relationship or the reinforcement contingency. Brewer (1974) cites five GSR studies which have used this 'masking' technique, and in each case the results show that there is no conditioning when the subject is unaware of the CS-UCS relationship.

Humphreys' (1939) classic study showed that intermittent CS-UCS pairings produced a conditioned response which was more resistant to extinction than the 100% pairings, and this result was explained in terms of expectancies; i. e. the intermittent reinforcement group took longer to become aware of the changed CS-UCS relationship during the extinction phase. On the other hand, Katz et al. (1971) found that subjects who had been exposed to variable levels of shock took very much longer than a constant-level 100% shock group to extinguish, *even though both groups had been clearly informed that no more shocks would occur*. The expectancy hypothesis is faced with some difficulties in explaining this result, and the cognitive position has not been immune from counterattack by S-R theorists.

Wolpe (1978) denied that cognitive variables function within a realm of activity independent from other sorts of stimuli. In Wolpe's view, cognition is ruled by the same lawfulness as other forms of behaviour, and his concept of imagery relies upon conditioning. The image is a conditioned perception, and thoughts are responses whether they are perceptions or imaginings. As such, they can be conditioned to other thoughts and to responses in other categories. Wolpe therefore includes cognitive variables within his system, but reclassifies them within a stimulus-response framework. In direct contrast to Brewer, Wolpe, who sees cognitive responses as a subset of behavioural responses, asserted that 'learning takes place automatically' (Wolpe 1978), and that neurotic anxiety is a response to definable aspects of the environment (Wolpe 1967b). Beech and Perigault (1974) use a similar sort of argument in their discussion of obsessional-compulsive neurosis, where they suggest that recurrent, intrusive and anxiety-evoking thoughts are usually elicited by environmental stimuli. The mental events have themselves acquired the properties of phobic stimuli in the same way as external stimuli (i. e. through conditioning).

With regard to the nature of psychological determinants, in Lewin's (1935) well-known formulation, behaviour was described as a function of personal and environmental variables: $B = f^{(P, E)}$. Bandura, however, questioned this on the grounds that personal and environmental factors do not operate independently; rather they determine each other. It is largely through their own actions that people produce the environmental conditions which surround them; and these in turn affect their behaviour. This relationship is described as *reciprocal determinism*. (The term 'reciprocal' is used here to mean mutual interaction between events, rather than in the more restricted sense of similar or opposite counter-reactions.) 'From the social learning perspective, psychological functioning is a continuous reciprocal interaction between the personal, behavioural, and environmental determinants' (Bandura 1977). In contrast to Lewin's formula, Bandura represents this as follows:

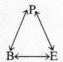

The relative strength of these factors varies with changing circumstances. At certain times, environmental factors will exert a powerful influence upon behaviour, whereas at other times personal factors will have the greatest impact.

The implications of this for the abnormal and clinical psychologist extend to the findings of Rosenhan (1973) about the effects of the social context upon the perception of 'abnormality'. In Rosenhan's study, eight pseudo-patients gained admission to 12 psychiatric hospitals in America by complaining of hearing voices: after admission they ceased simulating this symptom and behaved normally. All were diagnosed as either having a schizophrenic or a manic-depressive psychosis, and in none of the cases was the diagnosis reversed. Rosenhan found that the tendency to over-diagnose illness could be reversed by appropriate instructions, so that the psychiatric staff recognised pseudo-patients among the genuine patient group. In Rosenhan's view, the social context and the meanings attributed to the actions of the person labelled mentally ill are so powerful that they determine our perceptions of mental illness. In contrast to intrapsychic interpretations of neurosis, the social perspective extends the concept beyond the individual into his environment. It is recognised that the psychologist, psychiatrist and other members of staff play a large part in determining the regularities which are supposedly seen in mental illness (Ullmann and Krasner 1967).

The neurotic disorders cannot be reduced to objective, natural phenomena. Even if one were to regard the neuroses as illnesses in the full sense of the term (and few psychologists would accept this formulation), this remains true. From the psychological perspective, and particularly from a social and cognitive viewpoint, a neurotic disorder is best seen not merely as a behavioural response, but as a form of *social action*.

5.2 Modelling

Watson regarded the neurotic disorders as conditioned emotional responses produced by Pavlovian conditioning, and in Mowrer's two-stage theory, the initial conditioned fear response was explained in terms of classical conditioning. Eysenck (1976) has suggested that fear responses may be acquired by other means, for instance, through modelling or imitation learning, but S-R theorists have largely excluded these processes from their detailed analyses.

One of the first descriptions of the acquisition of fear as a result of social observation is that of Mary Cover Jones (1924), and more recently Marks (1969) described how fears may be acquired by this form of vicarious learning (variously called social learning, no-trial learning, vicarious conditioning, observational learning, modelling and imitation). Rachman (1977) continued to emphasise the importance of conditioning effects in the acquisition of fear and anxiety, but acknowledged the influence of two other determinants, both of which are indirect processes. The first, vicarious acquisition, relates to the work of Bandura and others on modelling. Rachman also suggested that fears may be acquired through the transmission of information or through instruction. Despite an almost complete absence of studies on this effect, it is clear that this sort of teaching is an inherent part of child-rearing. Parents, siblings and friends are all involved in this sort of interaction with children from their earliest years.

Church (1959) found that rats which had been shocked after observing other animals being shocked showed higher levels of fear to the pain of others than a control group which had received the same amount of aversive stimulation but unassociated with the pain responses of other animals. The same result has been obtained with other species, and Berger (1962) found that human subjects who observed another person being shocked would themselves show an emotional response to the initially neutral conditioned stimulus. Both Berger and Church discuss their results in terms of conditioning processes. Berger suggests that the observer's perceptions of the UCS and the performer's UCR are cues to the performer's unconditioned emotional response, and that this unconditioned response *as perceived by the observer* determines the oberserver's emotional response. This emphasis upon perception implies that the observer's emotional response may be based upon both correct and incorrect attributions.

Bandura (1971) assigns a more prominent role to cognition in this context. Modelling processes are said to operate principally through their informative function. The observer acquires mainly symbolic representations of the modelled events rather than specific S-R associations, and the observer functions as an active agent who transforms, classifies and organises the modelling stimuli into easily remembered schemes. Bandura suggests that the four components in observational learning are attentional processes, retention, motor-reproduction processes, and reinforcement and motivational effects. Vicarious aversive conditioning, for instance, is directly related to the degree of psychological stress in the observer (Bandura and Rosenthal 1966). There is, however, a point at which the level of arousal becomes so high that emotionality and vicarious conditioning become inversely related, and Bandura and Rosenthal interpreted their results in terms of an inverted-U relationship between arousal and vicarious conditioning.

Other investigations have shown that behavioural inhibitions can be acquired through observing aversive stimuli administered to performing subjects. In one study (Bandura 1965), a group of boys and girls (aged $3^1/_2$ to 6 years) watched a film of a model being aggressive towards a doll. In the model-rewarded condition, a second person complimented the model upon his behaviour and gave him such rewards as sweets and soft drinks. In the model-punished condition, the reinforcing agent strongly challenged the model's aggressive behaviour and physically punished him. The results showed that observing the reinforcing consequences for the model had a significant effect upon the behaviour that the children produced spontaneously after watching the film. There was also a highly significant difference between boys and girls. The boys developed more imitative aggression than the girls after exposure to an aggressive male model, though when offered a positive incentive to enact the aggressive behaviour, this sex difference practically disappeared. Bandura suggests that the sex differences in overt aggressive behaviour may primarily reflect a willingness to exhibit aggression, rather than any learning deficit. These findings support the view that responses may be inhibited or disinhibited as a result of observing the consequences of another person's behaviour.

There is evidence that phobic fears can be passed on from parents to children (Bandura 1969; Marks 1969). One young woman whose fear of spiders presented a marked social handicap appeared to have learned this from her family, in which a grandmother, mother, aunt and sister were all extremely afraid of spiders. The patient remembered that there was a bell in the house, and whenever a spider was seen the alarm was sounded and everyone ran screaming from the house.

In a study of 100 children with neurotic disorders, Britton (1969) looked at the incidence and severity of psychiatric disorders in their mothers. The children were allocated to three major groups according to their symptoms – *neurotic disorders* (anxiety, phobias, compulsions and mood disturbances), *conduct disorders* (lying, stealing etc.) and *mixed disorders,* in which both sorts of disturbance were present. Britton found no relationship between the presence or severity of psychiatric disorder in the mother and the type of disorder in the child. Only one symptom – separation anxiety – was related to the degree of maternal psychopathology. However, it was found that the children of neurotic and depressed mothers were most likely to show predominantly neurotic symptoms or combined neurotic and conduct disorders. Sixteen of the 21 children with neurotic or depressed mothers showed high levels of anxiety, whereas pathological anxiety was unusual in the children of mothers with personality disorders. There was also a significantly higher incidence of phobias and mood disorders among the children of neurotic and depressed mothers.

There is some disagreement between S-R theorists and social-cognitive theorists about the nature of the neurotic disorders and about anxiety itself. Although Wolpe (1970) has largely equated anxiety with autonomic arousal, this is a restrictive use of the concept.

Anxiety is best seen as a multidimensional concept which denotes a complex pattern of responses characterised by subjective apprehension, behavioural avoidance and autonomic arousal. These three components show some degree of independence (Rachman and Hodgson 1974), and a number of hypotheses relating to the notion of synchrony and desynchrony between the experiential, biological and behavioural components have been proposed by Hodgson and Rachman (1974); in particular they suggested that synchrony or desynchrony between the response systems is a function of the intensity of emotional arousal, level of demand, therapeutic technique and the specific physiological system which is being measured. Sartory et al. (1977) looked at these hypotheses and found some empirical support for them, though their results were in part inconclusive.

Borkovec (1976) also considered anxiety to involve any or all of these three separate but interacting response components, and there are nine possible relationships between them. Borkovec's analysis is interesting in that it specifies the sort of relationship which exists between the cognitive and physiological components of anxiety. When the immediate anxiety response involves a strong physiological component, cognitive factors will be relatively ineffective: simple manipulations of the cognitive and behavioural components will be more effective in those cases in which there is only a weak physiological component. However, Borkovec has pointed out how cognitive avoidance responses can maintain the physiological components of anxiety, and how many different cognitive manipulations (e. g. false feedback, misattribution, demand/expectancy effects and attention focusing) contribute towards the maintenance of anxiety.

5.3 Life Events and Neurosis

Psychological theories of neurosis, and particularly the conditioning theories, have tended to concentrate rather exclusively upon the individual and his specific learning experiences, to the neglect of the social circumstances in which the individual lives. Yet there is a well-documented relationship, for instance, between social class and the diagnosis of psychiatric disorder. In a series of studies in America, Hollingshead and Redlich (1958) found an inverse relationship between social class and the prevalence of psychosis (or the prevalence of diagnoses of psychosis, if one wishes to maintain an attitude of scepticism towards the validity of psychiatric diagnosis). The lower the social class, the higher was the prevalence of psychotic disorders; Hollingshead and Redlich found that the incidence of psychosis in social class 5 was three times higher than in social class 4.

These authors also reported a strong direct relationship between class status and the distribution of treated neuroses in the population. The effect of social class varied for each diagnostic group. 'Character neuroses' were most likely to be diagnosed in class 1 and 2 patients; and for depressive neuroses the rate declined almost in a straight line from class 1 to class 5. Antisocial reactions were most prevalent among class 3 patients, and hysterical reactions, unlike the other neurotic disorders, showed an inverse relationship with class position (being more prominent in class 5 patients). Hollingshead and Redlich described their concept of neurosis as 'a condition of subjective malaise and disturbed social interaction'. In addition, they regarded neurosis not only as a state of mind of the sufferer, but also as a result of the patient's interaction with the therapist, and suggested that the class positions of both therapist and patient may affect the resultant diagnosis.

It is likely that an important feature of this interaction is the patient's attitudes toward the 'neurotic' label. He may accept or reject this attribution according to his own or other people's appraisal of his behaviour and personality, and the criteria for assumption of the neurotic role probably differ from class to class. Hollingshead and Redlich's data, for instance, suggest that there are differences between the readiness of the various social classes to accept the 'patient' self-concept which depend on (a) degree of discomfort, (b) whether one's body hurts or functions poorly, (c) being unable to work properly, (d) interpersonal difficulties and (e) difficulties with the law. In this way, a neurotic disorder is an important part of each person's definition of his class position in society and expresses an attitude towards the way he expects to be able to function.

There is also a sizeable body of research which has been concerned with the relationship between socially stressful life events and mental health. The concept of social stress is rather vague, and Coates et al. (1976) have described four different ways in which the term is used:

1) Stress as background; this includes the sort of living conditions and social supports that are available to an individual.
2) Stress as the pace of life, including the pressure and intensity of daily life. When stress is interpreted in these terms, life events are significantly related to high levels of anxiety, concern over one's health and personal distress (Coates et al. 1969). Other definitions of social stress have included –
3) Stress as changes in the pace of life.
4) Stress as acceleration in the rate of living.

These sorts of stress also have some effect on mental health. It is well known that emigration, bereavement, personal illness and natural disasters can have an adverse effect on the mental health of some individuals.

One of the more sophisticated studies of the effects of social stress and life events upon psychological health is that of Brown and Harris (1978). In contrast to Hollingshead and Redlich's study, their own investigation of depression in women showed that in London, psychiatric disorder, and depression in particular, was more common amongst working class women. Brown and Harris emphasised the view of depression as a social phenomenon and, in explaining their findings, used a model similar to that in Fig. 5. This describes how a depressive reaction results from the interaction of social class, protective and vulnerability factors and specific stressful events (the provoking agents). The provoking agents determine when the depression occurs, and the vulnerability factors determine whether or not these agents will have an effect. In addition, Brown and Harris proposed that a class of symptom-formation factors (not shown in Fig. 5) also operate to determine the severity and form of the depressive disorder. A major loss in the past, for instance, particularly in childhood or adolescence, is seen as the most potent factor influencing the severity of depression; it was suggested that the loss of a mother before age 11 significantly increased the risk of depression in adulthood, whereas the same loss between ages 11 and 17 had no influence.

Although many studies have cited correlational findings which suggest that social class and the prevalence of certain psychological disorders may be related in some way, there has been little explicit discussion of the nature of this relationship. Brown and Harris's study is valuable because of the way in which it attempts this sort of analysis. As well as social class, they took into account five 'life stages' related to the age of the women and the age of their youngest child. Among the working-class subjects, the highest rate of

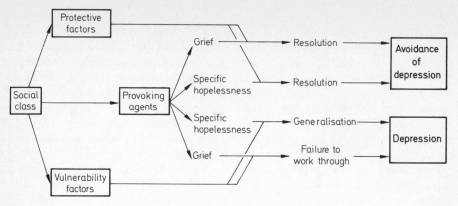

Fig. 5

psychiatric disorder (the majority of these being cases of depression) was found among women with a child of under 6 years. Middle-class women showed no differences in terms of life stage, and there was no class difference in the risk of becoming depressed among women without children. When they looked at the different types of life events which happened to their different groups, Brown and Harris found that severe household events were more likely to occur amongst women with children and that for these events there was a class difference; working-class women were three times more likely to have at least one severe household event. Among the events included in this category, Brown and Harris cite the following: being given a month's notice at a long-standing job, husband losing his job, son in trouble with police, husband sent to prison, being threatened with eviction, etc.

It was also found that the difficulties faced by working-class women tended to last longer than for middle-class subjects. The results showed that among women with children who have had a severe event or a major difficulty, 31% of the working-class women developed depression compared with 8% of middle-class women.

Among their depressed subjects, Brown and Harris found that almost all had a severe event or some other provoking factor. However, only one-fifth of those with such provoking agents broke down. In order to explain this, the authors invoked the notion of vulnerability and protective factors. One of the most significant protective factors was the presence of an intimate and confiding relationship with a friend or relative (usually a husband or boy-friend). Again, it was suggested that working-class women were more vulnerable than middle-class women; as well as being less likely to have a husband as a confidant, working-class women were also more likely to have lost a mother and to have three or more children younger than 14 at home.

5.4 Labelling

Although Brown and Harris are sociologists, their work incorporates a number of important psychological and psychiatric concepts as well as the social and sociological ones. The S-R theorists have generally defined neurosis in terms of maladaptive behaviour;

they have not, however, been particularly concerned to explore this aspect of behaviour in any depth. Indeed, one sociological criticism of behaviour modification is that in practice it often operates in the same way as the medical model, as an individual system of mental disorder. Scheff (1966) argued that the techniques of behaviour modification are oriented towards changing the patient's psychological system rather than the interpersonal or social system of which he is a member, and this tends to isolate the symptom from its context. Although Scheff's criticism may be appropriate in some cases, it is probably over-stated. It is not clear, for instance, why it should be *necessary* for a behaviour therapist to change the social environment of a patient with fears of contamination and obsessional-compulsive rituals, though in some cases the treatment of obsessions may be facilitated if it is extended into the patient's home environment and involves the patient's relatives (Marks 1973 a–b). In some cases of neurosis, the disorder may be an individual one: in other cases, the therapist ignores the social context at his own, and at his patient's, peril. As illustrations of this one might cite drug addiction, alcoholism, fetishism, homosexuality, reactive depression and probably many agoraphobic and hysterical disorders. In sociological terms, such behaviours may be regarded as deviance and as the violation of social norms which leads to negative social sanctions; in these terms an important function of the social model of mental disorder is to provide a framework which avoids the questionable assumptions of *inherent* psychopathology in all cases of neurosis.

In their assertion that mental illness may be seen as an ascribed social role, the sociological critics do have some psychological company. Ullmann and Krasner (1969) have described a social role in the terminology of operant conditioning, as a category of instrumental acts which are reinforced in a given situation. Specific roles, such as that of father, lecturer or patient, include those elements of behaviour which are common to certain specific types of situation, and the individual behaves in the way which is most likely to produce some reward. The performance of a particular role depends upon the individual's past experiences and his ability to perform the role. Neurotic behaviour is maladaptive in its failure to meet the expectations held by the patient and/or by others for someone in his role.

In an investigation of women receiving state welfare payments, Cole and Lejeune (1977) found that 45% of their subjects complained of 'nerves', and that defining one's health as poor was associated with emotional complaints. The authors suggested that many welfare mothers regarded their welfare status as a kind of personal failure and were prone to adopt the sick-role as a justification of their failure. Those women who regarded themselves as inadequate wives and mothers were particularly likely to define their health as poor. These results demonstrate the important interaction of the individual's self-perceptions (possibly acting as the protective factors suggested by Brown and Harris) and their social circumstances.

Few psychologists, and even fewer psychiatrists, would be prepared to go quite so far as the societal-reactance theorists and assert that the maladaptive behaviour which causes a person to become labelled as 'neurotic' has little relationship to the personal and social attributes of the individual. Lemert (1967), however, has suggested that primary deviance (in this case, the neurotic behaviour itself) 'has only marginal implications for the psychic structure of the individual.' This is essentially the same position as that of Scheff (1966), who also regarded mental illness as an ascribed status dependent mainly upon conditions external to the individual.

Others have found a different pattern. Yarrow et al. (1955) looked at the ways in which wives came to regard their husbands as mentally ill. They found that the wives showed a marked resistance to interpreting the husband's behaviour as 'ill' rather than 'normal', and it was only when his behaviour exceeded tolerable limits that the wife sought medical help. Even at this point the wife would often resist seeing the behaviour as illness. Gove (1970) cites a number of studies which reach this same conclusion – that the psychological disturbance occurs prior to the process of labelling rather than as a consequence of it.

According to the societal-reaction theory, the experience of being caught and labelled as a deviant is a crucial stage in the development of deviant behaviour, and this is largely related to the person's position in the social structure. The greater an individual's social and economic resources, the greater his chances of being able to deal successfully with others and therefore avoid being channelled into a socially deviant role. In the case of the psychological disorders, this implies that the higher an individual's social status, the more likely he is to avoid treatment and particularly in-patient treatment. This is broadly in agreement with Hollingshead and Redlich's (1958) data on psychotic disorders, and the results of Brown and Harris's (1978) study on depression could also be interpreted in this light. On the other hand, in an investigation of 258 in-patients which examined the predictions of societal reaction theory, Gove and Howell (1974) found that the resources of the individual generally appear to facilitate entrance into psychiatric treatment, including in-patient treatment. This is contrary to what one would expect on the basis of the societal-reaction account. However, Gove and Howell are careful to point out that their results do not imply that the processes suggested by the societal-reaction account do not exist, but that they are not usually the most salient effects.

Gove (1975) has also challenged the suggestion that those individuals who have been labelled 'mentally ill' have undergone a profound and generally irreversible change. Rosenhan (1973) referred to the labelling process in order to account for the ways in which psychiatric patients are perceived by staff. Rosenhan suggested that the psychiatric label profoundly colours the perception of other people towards the patient, and that the distortion is often great enough to lead the staff to overlook or misinterpret normal behaviour. It is true that the public stereotype of mental illness is often inaccurate and distorted. The psychiatric patient is often regarded with fear, distrust and dislike, and this negative stereotype of the mentally ill is probably shared by many professionals. But although this view of the mentally ill is negative and suggestive of serious discrimination, data on the effects of social stigmatisation after being treated in a psychiatric hospital are fairly sparse. Gove and Fain (1973) found no evidence of deterioration in the occupational status, social relationships or financial situation of a group of patients after hospitalisation. If anything, their results suggested a slight improvement. Most of the patients themselves saw their stay in hospital as having been beneficial and felt that their ability to handle problems had improved: only a small number felt that the stigma associated with hospitalisation had proved a serious problem for them. This study suggests that when dealing with someone who has been mentally ill, most people do not seriously discriminate against them. Although labelling processes may have some effect, societal reaction theorists have over-emphasised the importance of such factors in the explanation of psychological disorder, and parts of the societal-reaction account of mental illness seem to be substantially incorrect. However, its greatest value to psychological medicine may be that it draws attention to a much neglected facet of psychological disorders and helps to correct the predominantly individualistic bias of most psychologists and psychiatrists.

5.5 Attribution

One area of research in social and cognitive psychology that is directly relevant to any theory of neurosis is that concerning attribution. The term 'interpersonal attribution' refers to the process or processes by which we come to attribute various dispositions, motives, intentions, abilities and responsibilities to one another (and indeed to one's own behaviour). Attributions are a sort of explanation of *why* someone acted as he did and assume that people are active agents, capable, at least in principle, of free and intentional action and of determining their own behaviour (Eiser 1978).

In their classic experiment, Schachter and Singer (1962) showed how an individual's emotions were dependent both upon physiological arousal and upon environmental cues which might account for the arousal. After receiving an injection of adrenalin or a placebo injection of saline solution, one-third of the subjects were correctly informed of the drug effects, one-third were incorrectly informed, and the third group received no information. When the subjects then encountered another person who acted in an angry or euphoric manner, the subjects who had received the injection of adrenalin and who had no clear explanation as to their own arousal were most likely to be influenced by their social circumstances. They tended to behave in a similar manner to the experimental confederate. The subjects who had been correctly informed of the reasons for their aroused state were able to attribute this to the drug effect and were uninfluenced by the emotional behaviour of the actor. Subsequent research showed that a person's emotionality could be decreased by falsely attributing an emotional state to a non-emotional source (Nisbett and Schachter 1966).

The implications of this research suggest that emotions, and specifically pathological emotional states, may be significantly affected by the attributions that a person makes about the causes of his neurotic symptomatology. Storms and Nisbett (1970) looked at the way in which attribution processes could affect the emotional behaviour of insomniacs. Subjects were given placebo tablets; one group was told that the drugs would lead to insomniac effects, i. e. that they would cause alertness, increased heart rate and increased body temperature. The other group was informed that their drugs were sedatives. The authors hypothesised that the subjects who had received the 'stimulant' drug would be able to reattribute their sleeplessness to the drug and therefore would experience less emotional arousal and fall asleep more quickly. The other group, having received a supposedly sedative drug, might have been expected to attribute their sleeplessness to personal causes and to experience greater insomnia. (This is, incidentally, quite the opposite prediction to that made on the basis of a 'suggestibility' model.) The results showed that subjects' attributions about their symptoms influenced the subsequent intensity of their emotional states. Those subjects who had taken 'stimulants' reported a decrease in the time that it took them to fall asleep, whereas the 'sedative' group took longer.

Storms and Nisbett also interviewed the subjects after the study and found that the subjects' accounts of their insomnia were consistent with an attributional model. It was notable that each of the subjects had adopted the label of 'insomniac' and believed that this carried with it the further implications of some special psychological condition. Many also described their difficulties in falling asleep in the following terms. After going to bed they would begin to look for signs of insomnia, such as feeling too hot or being easily disturbed and upset by noise; having noticed these, they would feel anxious and begin to imagine the consequences the next day of another sleepless night. This would increase their anxieties and keep them awake, perhaps speculating on the underlying causes of their difficulties, which would in turn increase their level of anxiety even further.

This description has close parallels to the anxiety-feedback cycle which was described by Eysenck (1975b) as a possible cause of such disorders as impotence and insomnia, though the explanation offered by Eysenck is quite different. Storms and Nisbett use a more explicitly cognitive and attributional framework to account for their results, the key elements being self-attributions of pathology or inadequacy, and increased anxiety. Like Eysenck, they too suggest that their analysis may apply to such disorders as male impotence, stuttering, extreme shyness and excessive physical awkwardness. Valins and Nisbett (1971) have extended this analysis to other neurotic disorders, such as depression, homosexual panic and phobic disorders. In many of these cases the person becomes aware of their own problems at the symptomatic level before seeking professional advice from a therapist. In doing so, they often reach self-diagnoses of abnormality or inadequacy that can set up the vicious cycle of increased anxiety and increased difficulties. Such self-attributions are probably found in most neurotic patients and may present a severe obstacle to therapeutic change.

Storms and McCaul (1976) discussed the evidence for this two-stage process. Their review suggested that the level of experienced anxiety is directly related both to the individual's attributions of control over his environment and to situational stress factors. To the extent that he feels helpless or out of control, he is likely to experience considerable anxiety, and these self-cognitions can interact with external factors to produce magnified increases in anxiety. In insomnia and male impotence, there is evidence that excessive arousal of the sympathetic nervous system is directly related to the problem (e. g. Monroe 1967; Masters and Johnson 1970). In other cases, however, the relationship between the anxiety and the disorder is likely to be cognitively mediated.

In an investigation of the effects of attributional processes upon stuttering, Storms and McCaul (1976) found that normal speakers who were led to make a dispositional attribution for their speech faults (pauses, repetitions, stammers, etc.) found it more difficult to perform a verbal task under conditions of stress than other subjects who were given a situational explanation of their speech faults. In this case, the results support the suggestion that dispositional attributions interact with higher levels of stress to produce an exacerbation of stammering. Negative self-attributions may also play an important role in producing the more severe speech difficulties that lead individuals to seek therapeutic assistance (Storms and McCaul 1976).

In therapy, it has been suggested that individuals who have developed *dispositional* explanations of their behaviour may be helped if the therapist helps them to substitute *situational* attributions. This distinction between intrinsic and extrinsic causes of behaviour is of fundamental importance to the application of attribution theory to clinical practice. Valins and Nisbett (1972) discussed some of the ways in which attribution processes effect the development and treatment of emotional disorders, but as a comparatively recent research topic, there ic clearly a need for further investigations of what appears to be a promising area for clinical research.

5.6 Cognitive Accounts of Depression

One of the unfortunate consequences of the medical model is that psychological disorders have tended to be seen as distinct and different from normal forms of behaviour. So whereas social psychology has investigated the relationship between cognition and emotion (e. g. Schachter and Singer 1962), psychiatry has frequently preserved the concept of depression as a primary affective disorder in which cognitive factors play little part. Any cognitive abnormalities in depressive disorders have usually been seen as the inevitable result of affective distortions, possibly due to the disorganisation that can follow intense emotions.

Beck (1971) pointed out how this notion of the primacy of affect over cognition in psychopathology is contrary to that which applies for normal subjects. Here, the way a person sees his situation determines his affective state, and Beck has argued that the direction of the reaction is exactly the same in the depressive disorders. The difference between the normal and abnormal reactions is to be found in the degree of correspondence between the cognition and reality. In the abnormal condition, there is a distorted cognitive representation of reality, and in the case of the depressed patient, the cognitions show a *systematic error* (biased against the person's own interests).

The thought content of neurotic depressive patients often centres around what Beck calls 'the cognitive triad' – a negative self-image, a negative view of life's experiences and a nihilistic view of the future. The typical emotions of depression, sadness, disappointment and apathy follow from the sense of loss, negative expectations and helplessness (Beck 1971). A similar discussion has been offered by Melges and Bowlby (1969), who stressed the central role played by attitudes in many psychological disorders and in particular by feelings of hopelessness and the anticipation of failure. Melges and Bowlby suggested that a key process in depression is the belief that available plans of action can no longer achieve established goals.

Seligman has also described a theory of depression based upon the notion of learned helplessness, in which cognitions of helplessness operate as the basic cause of depression (Seligman 1975). Seligman's account is an important development in the psychology of depression, since it is the first full-scale treatment of the issue which starts from an experimental rather a clinical point of view. Although both are cognitive accounts of depression, Seligman's theory differs from that of Beck in its denial of the value of distinguishing between cognition and emotion in this context. In depression there is an interdependence of feelings and thought; a person does not feel depressed without depressing thoughts, nor does he have depressing thoughts without feeling depressed.

Seligman pointed out how the subject in a Pavlovian conditioning experiment is helpless; his responses have no effect upon the CS and UCS, whereas in operant conditioning, the subject's voluntary response controls the outcome. Overmier and Seligman (1967) found that dogs which had been exposed to inescapable shock in a Pavlovian harness were unable to learn an escape/avoidance response in a shuttle box as effectively as animals without this experience of inescapable shock. Typically, the animals exposed to uncontrollable shock did not escape from the shock in the shuttle box, but passively accepted the shock. When the experimental animals had first received escapable shock in the shuttle box, then inescapable shock in the harness, they did not react passively to shock when they were again placed in the shuttle box, as did animals which had first received inescapable shock in the shuttle box (Seligman and Maier 1967). Seligman suggests that when an organism has had an initial experience of uncontrollable trauma, its motivation to respond to later trauma is likely to wane.

In a study with rats, Seligman and Meyer (1970) found that animals which received unpredictable high-intensity shocks when bar-pressing for food reduced their response levels to about 10% of the pre-shock rate, and that this suppression appeared to be permanent. At the end of a 70-day period, no recovery was evident. Animals which were exposed to low levels of shock, or to predictable shock, did not show this same suppression. It was also found in this experiment that stomach and intestinal ulceration were significantly more likely to occur in the fearful (response-suppression) animals. Seligman has used a safety-signal hypothesis to explain these results – that after experiences of trauma, an organism will remain in fear unless it is in the presence of a signal which reliably predicts safety. In this formulation, fear is a joint function of the intensity of shock and the probability that shock will occur.

Seligman's results with respect to stomach ulcers and uncontrollability are quite different from those of Brady. In what became a classic experiment, Brady et al. (1958) divided a group of monkeys into pairs. Each animal received a shock unless one of the pair, the 'executive' monkey, pressed a lever which delayed the shock for both animals. After a period of weeks, several 'executive' animals died, and analysis showed extensive gastro-intestinal lesions with ulceration in the experimental animals but not in the controls. These results were interpreted to show that it was the decision-making animals who developed the psychosomatic disorders, and not the animals who received uncontrollable shock. However, there is a serious methodological drawback to Brady's study. This concerns selection of animals for the experimental and control conditions. Brady's animals were not randomly assigned to the 'executive' and helplessness conditions. During the initial session, those animals which first showed avoidance lever-pressing to delay the shock were chosen to be the 'executive' animal. It is possible that these animals learned avoidance responses more quickly because they were more emotional, and therefore more susceptible to stomach ulcers, in which case, Brady's result would be an artifact of his experimental design – a possibility which is admitted by the authors.

Seligman's helplessness theory of depression is intended to account for three facets of the disorder; disturbances of motivation, emotion and cognition. In its simplest form, it suggests that when an organism is faced by an outcome which is independent of its responses, as for instance in classical conditioning, it learns that the outcome is independent of the responses made (Seligman 1975). Put in these terms, this seems so obvious as to be hardly worth stating. However, a non-cognitive learning theory faces some problems in accounting for learnt expectancies about the probability of any given outcome. Seligman's theory starts with information about the response-outcome contingency, then moves to a *cognitive representation* of the contingency and finally to the behavioural response. When the outcome is independent of any response the person makes, Seligman predicts that this will establish a belief or expectation about the inefficacy of responding and difficulty in learning that success can follow responding. When the uncontrollable outcome is also traumatic, such conditions will produce heightened anxiety followed by depression.

There have been objections to the learned helplessness model on both empirical and theoretical grounds, and Abramson et al. (1978) proposed a reformulated account that incorporates the individual's attributions. The person first learns that his responses and certain outcomes are independent and then makes an attribution about the cause of these events.

In one of the Glass and Singer studies (1972), subjects were exposed to a loud noise. Those subjects who were able to turn off this noise performed better in a problem-solving task than others who were unable to avoid the noise. However, another group of subjects was told that they could turn the noise off if they wanted to, but that the experimenters preferred that they did not do so. In fact, these subjects were unable to stop the noise, but *believed* that they could control it. Under these conditions, they performed as well as the subjects who actually did turn off the noise. Actual controllability and actual uncontrollability can produce identical expectations; it is the cognitive representation of the world that is the crucial determinant of helplessness. It is also possible (and clinically, it may be quite common) for a person to believe incorrectly that environmental events are uncontrollable when they could be controlled. A person may for several reasons be unable to find an appropriate coping response for a particular situation and therefore believe that he is unable to control events.

But despite the introduction of attribution into the model, it remains vulnerable. There are a number of conceptual difficulties still inherent in the theory. Buchwald et al. (1978) criticised the indiscriminate use of the notion of learned helplessness to refer to observed interference with performance, to specific deficits that might have caused the interference, and to the belief that responses and their outcomes are independent. When this ambiguous usage is linked to the complex and heterogeneous collection of signs and symptoms that comprise clinical depression, the possibilities of confusion multiply.

On empirical grounds there are other difficulties. Of the three experiments of Willis and Blaney (1978), none gave clear support to the predictions made by the helplessness model. Other studies found that some subjects react to conditions of uncontrollability by renewed determination and effort. This apparently paradoxical facilitation effect was reported by Hanusa and Schulz (1977), and by Wortman et al. (1976). Indeed, these studies found the facilitation effect in those conditions that the revised helplessness model predicts would lead to the strongest deficits (i. e. where subjects were led to attribute their failure to their own lack of ability). Wortman and Dintzer (1978) point out that unless it is possible to specify in advance that certain attributions will be followed by specific consequences, the model falls into circularity.

5.7 Social Anxiety and Social Competence

Neither the ICD-8 nor DSM-II classification systems differentiate between the varieties of phobic disorder that occur. Marks (1970), however, distinguished between agoraphobic disorders, social phobias, situational and animal phobias, and the revised American system DSM-III is to include social phobias within the general category of anxiety disorders. Social phobias are said to be characterised by a fear of situations in which the person is exposed to possible scrutiny by others and in which he might behave badly. The person with a social phobia is likely to show marked anticipatory anxiety if required to enter such situations and to avoid them. The diagnostic criteria for social phobia are primarily the avoidance of specific social situations, and the distress which is a result of that avoidance.

One of the difficulties with this concept of social phobia is that the phobic disorders are essentially linked to particular objects or events, whereas in this case the social fears are often so generalised that it is difficult to specify what is acting as the socially phobic stimulus. To this extent, the term 'social phobia' may be misleading, and in the present discussion the term 'social anxiety' is preferred as a descriptive label, since it contains less surplus meaning. Of course the term 'phobia' itself varies in its meaning: Eysenck and Rachman (1965) have used it as if it were synonymous with conditioned emotional response, whereas in Freudian theory it implies displacement. In Marks' (1970) view, phobias are intense fears which are out of proportion to the apparent stimulus, which cannot be reasoned away, and which lead to avoidance of the feared stimulus.

In one discussion of severe social anxiety (Nichols 1974), 12 separate aspects of this disorder were described. The first was a sensitivity to, and fearfulness of, disapproval and criticism. It is an important feature of Zajonc's (1965) notion of social facilitation that the presence of others, in the role of observers or of co-participants, leads to a state of generalised arousal. More recent research suggests that the presence of others is, in itself, largely irrelevant; it is the possibility of being evaluated by them that produces the apprehension (Cottrell et al. 1968). This effect is most marked when the audience is seen as likely to be destructively critical and least marked when the audience is seen as a source of help. In other words, the effect of other people depends largely upon whether they are seen as safety-signals or threat-signals. As yet there is no clear statement of the precise conditions under which audiences produce increased or decreased levels of anxiety, though Nichols (1974) suggested that the highly socially anxious person may tend to see criticism where in reality there is none. Among the other features described by Nichols are low self-evaluation, anticipatory fears of failure in social situations, rigid concepts of appropriate social behaviour and fears of being seen by others as behaving oddly. These cognitive aspects of severe social anxiety have been largely neglected by psychological accounts of the phobic and neurotic disorders.

The increasing interest in the psychology of interpersonal behaviour (e. g. Argyle 1969) has prompted a greater interest among clinical psychologists in social-training techniques as a form of therapy, and Mahoney (1974) has described a shift in behaviour-treatment research from a focus upon discrete, situation-specific responses and problem-specific procedures towards a more general coping-skills model. Social incompetence has usually been equated with the degree of subjective dissatisfaction felt by an individual in the performance of required social roles, which leads to an avoidance of these roles. Argyle et al. (1974) suggested that some forms of mental disorder are caused or exacerbated by lack of social competence and can be cured or alleviated by social-skills training programmes.

Depressed individuals may show such deficits as poor verbal behaviour (of a flat, passive and expressionless kind), lack of initiative in conversation and little interest in maintaining friendships or an active social life. Anxious patients, on the other hand, often show their anxiety in rapid, breathy speech which seems to come out under pressure, by a tense posture and jerky and poorly co-ordinated gestures. Among the other social-skills deficits that are sometimes found among individuals with neurotic disorders are disturbed perceptions of their own and other people's actions, and aggressive and hostile reactions to others. Patients with more severe disorders, such as schizophrenia, may be correspondingly more disturbed in their social behaviour.

Until recently there was comparatively little interest in, or knowledge about, the elements and processes of social behaviour, and even less was known about how these might fail. The social-skills model proposed by Trower et al. (1978) assumes that skills are acquired through various forms of learning, such as imitation, reinforcement and instruction, and through exposure to skilled models, and the authors include the following non-verbal elements in their discussion of social skills: facial expression, bodily gestures, gaze, spacial behaviour, non-verbal aspects of speech, bodily contact and physical appearance. The social functions of speech include giving instructions or directions which are intended to influence the behaviour of others directly, asking questions either to elicit an appropriate reply or to initiate an encounter, and offering comments or suggestions. Speech is also used to express emotions or attitudes, and it is used in informal chat in which little information is exchanged. Some verbal behaviour has a formal function, such as giving speeches or engaging in a socially routine interaction (greetings, farewells, thanks, etc.), and it is also possible to look at speech in terms of the latent and implicit messages which it contains.

Social-skills training is, necessarily, a complex package of interventions which is likely to vary from therapist to therapist, and even from occasion to occasion. In its simplest form, the training might begin with an assessment procedure designed to identify the specific types of social difficulties faced by the individual, who is then encouraged gradually to try out unaccustomed forms of behaviour. This often begins with careful observation of the circumstances of particular social situations, cautious interaction in the role, at first of a listener and then in a more active participation as a speaker. With increasing confidence the client is encouraged to try out more ambitious interactions by the use of assertive and rewarding strategies.

Because of the complexity both of the training procedures and of the social difficulties being treated, there have been considerable difficulties in conducting adequate evaluative research studies of these sorts of intervention. Wolpe (1958) reported that assertiveness training was an effective treatment for a group of out-patients with neurotic difficulties, and Hallam (1974) used social-skills training together with an extinction schedule to eliminate the performance of obsessional rituals. In a study of 20 patients, Trower et al. (1978) found that after ten individual sessions there were significant reductions in symptoms of anxiety, depression and social anxiety: the authors also suggested that social-skills training was superior to desensitisation procedures in dealing with specific, rather than general, difficulties. Marzillier (1978) concluded that skills training can improve behavioural skills, that the effects of training can generalise to real life and can be of lasting benefit, and that such training programmes are of clinical benefit to the patient.

5.8 Further Implications for Therapy

Meichenbaum (1976, 1977) has adopted a therapeutic policy which is based both on the cognitive work of Beck, Kelley, Singer and others, and upon more conventional behaviour-therapy research. This *cognitive-behaviour modification* assumes that any distinction between a purely behavioural versus a cognitive therapeutic programme is misleading and mistaken, and it has been suggested that the common basis of therapeutic change, regardless of the persuasions of the therapist, lies in the alteration of the internal dialogue in which the person engages (Meichenbaum 1976).

It is one of Meichenbaum's criticisms of clinical research that not enough attention has been paid to what happens in therapy prior to the beginning of specific treatments (e. g. a behaviour-modification programme). In some ways this is a similar complaint to that of Ramsay (1975), who discussed the question of the client's motivation for treatment. In a study of individuals who suffered from phobic disorders, Ramsay found that only a low percentage chose to enter therapy for their problems, and of these, many were probably only marginally motivated. In his actual clinical practise, Ramsay pointed out that despite the effectiveness of behaviour therapy as a treatment for phobias, much of his time was spent not in using the techniques themselves, but in bolstering the motivation of the patient to stay in treatment so that the techniques could be given a chance to work. This issue of the patient's motivation to co-operate with the therapist is of crucial importance in most areas of psychological medicine. Clinicians will recognise the problem from their own experience, yet it has received hardly any mention in the literature, and as a concept, it has often been misused. In the treatment of drug dependence, for instance, therapeutic failures have been excused on the grounds of the patient's lack of motivation rather than the inadequacy of the treatment. But despite the dangers of tautologous thinking involved in this misuse of the term, motivation for treatment can be rescued from circularity if it is related to the patient's perceptions and expectations prior to treatment (Gossop 1978c).

One theme of cognitive-behaviour modification is that the original S-R conceptualisation of behaviour therapy over-emphasised the importance of environmental events (antecedents and consequences), to the neglect of the individual's perceptions and evaluations of these events. Meichenbaum and Cameron (1974) reviewed the empirical evidence relating to this proposition; they concluded that when standard behaviour-therapy procedures were augmented with self-instructional components designed to help modify the client's cognitions, the treatment effects were more powerful, showed greater generalisation and lasted longer.

Meichenbaum's (1976) discussion of cognitive factors in behaviour-modification programmes examined the role of the client's expectations in therapy. It is clearly important that both client and therapist should have a common view of what they are doing. In this conceptualisation phase of treatment, an attempt is made to have the client change his perceptions, attributions and sense of control or helplessness about his presenting difficulties. It has been suggested that faulty self-evaluations are at the root of many adult neurotic disorders. One of the best-known statements of this position is Albert Ellis' *rational emotive therapy* (1957, 1962). Ellis proposed that a major core of emotional disturbances is a result of the individual's preoccupation with what others think of him. The aims of the therapist are centred upon making the client aware of his negative self-statements and of the anxiety-provoking and self-defeating nature of this sort of thinking. Meichenbaum (1976) has also emphasised the therapeutic significance of the patient's internal dialogue about his own difficulties and has attempted to modify this internal dialogue. Meichenbaum has described this as a three-stage process. In stage 1 the client is taught to become an observer of his own behaviour; this is then used as a stimulus for the person to emit different cognitions and behaviours; finally, the internal dialogue that the person has about his newly acquired behaviour determines whether or not the change will be maintained and will generalise. Both Ellis and Meichenbaum are primarily interested in the therapeutic implications of this position, and it has been suggested that whether or not the patient actually engaged in this sort of internal dialogue prior to therapy is less important than his willingness to view his behaviour *as if* it were affected by his self-statements and modifiable by them (Meichenbaum 1977). To this extent, the self-verbalisation hypothesis is more appropriately regarded as a therapeutic strategy than an explanation of the development of emotional disturbances.

The research into modelling effects has also had an impact upon treatment. It has been shown that behavioural inhibitions and conditioned emotional responses can be acquired by observers after watching the actions of another person and the consequences of those actions for the model (e. g. Bandura 1977; Berger 1962). It has also been suggested that established avoidance responses can be extinguished vicariously. Bandura et al. (1967) found that children who had observed a confident model gradually perform increasingly fear-provoking acts showed a marked and persistent reduction in their own avoidance behaviour.

Rachman (1972) looked at the clinical potential of the research findings on observational learning and concluded that the fear/anxiety reducing value of therapeutic modelling has been convincingly demonstrated. Symbolic modelling (in which the observer watches, but has no direct contact with either the therapist or the situation) produced a significant and lasting reduction of fear, and participant modelling increased the extent of the fear reduction. Modelling is not, however, a necessary condition for therapeutic change, since some methods produce successful results in the absence of any modelling experiences.

It is not clear, however, what the basis for these results is. One possibility is that the modelling conveys information to the observer about the probable outcomes of close interactions with feared stimuli (in this case, dogs). On the other hand, the reduction in avoidance behaviour could be due to extinction processes following the non-occurrence of the expected aversive consequences. Bandura (1969, 1977) suggested that the information derived from observing a model can be stored and used later as symbolic cues to overt behaviour.

Rachman (1972) suggested that modelling, desensitisation and flooding may each be based upon some common underlying process, possibly extinction, since in each form of treatment, the patient is exposed for extended periods of time to the fear-provoking stimuli. It is also possible that habituation of reinforcement effects could underlie these procedures, though it is difficult to explain the effectiveness of symbolic modelling in terms of reinforcement effects, since no response is made during the modelling period which could be reinforced.

The theoretical basis for the effects of modelling are not clear. Nonetheless, the practical effectiveness of modelling procedures has established their place in the clinical work of many therapists, and it seems likely that modelling will come to play an increasingly important role in the treatment of a wide range of neurotic and social disorders.

The therapeutic implications of the learned-helplessness model of depression have been presented by Abramson et al. (1978). The therapist might assist the depressed patient by helping them: (1) to change the probability of aversive events (e. g. by the use of social agencies to achieve rehousing or job-placement); (2) to re-evaluate the outcome itself (e. g. by substituting realistic goals for unrealistic ones); (3) to change their expectation from one of helplessness and uncontrollability to controllability (e. g. through social-skills training); and (4) to change their attributions of success and failure. Abramson et al. suggest that the person's attributions may be changed through discussion, though there is little evidence that cognitions can be changed quite so simply. There are, however, several studies that suggest that cognitive treatments for depression can be more effective than either anti-depressant medication (Rush et al. 1977) or behaviour therapy (Shaw 1977). In view of the current popularity of this model, further studies can be confidently expected to extend our understanding of its therapeutic potential.

6. Psycho-analytic Theories of Neurosis

Psycho-analysis – that interesting but peculiar and arcane doctrine: it has received more publicity and it has had more impact upon child-rearing, psychiatric training, art and literature than any other psychological theory, yet in any precise form it manages to remain obscure. Of all the theories presented in this book, it is perhaps the furthest from common-sense psychology, and yet its impact upon the layman has been so great that it is often mistakenly thought to constitute the whole of psychology.

It is difficult to provide any complete account of the psycho-analytic theories of neurosis within a chapter of this length. Even if one equated psycho-analysis with Freud's own work, it would be impossible to achieve such an aim. Freud's collected works alone run to 24 volumes in their English translation, and within these works he distinguished between several different meanings of the concept of neurosis and developed several different theories to explain the neurotic disorders.

Indeed, because Freud said so many different things at different times as his theory evolved, it has been suggested that only an historical account of the development of his ideas can provide a proper framework for understanding Freudian psychology (Nagera 1969).

When the various analytic factions that dissociated themselves (in varying degrees) from Freud's views are also taken into account, the problem assumes an even more daunting aspect. For these reasons the present chapter offers a necessarily selective review of Freud's writings on the neuroses, with emphasis upon certain of the key issues in his work. The chapter deals mainly with the Freudian system, since this provides a prototype of the psycho-analytic approach, though a brief description is also offered of some of the theoretical criticisms and modifications of classical Freudian theory made by other influential analysts.

6.1 Psychological Determinism

One of the most general aspects of Freud's attempt to understand human psychology was the tenet that human behaviour is never 'accidental'. Whereas other psychologists might have believed that the small mistakes of everyday life, dreams, jokes and so forth might ultimately be dependent on a complex interaction of certain laws of behaviour, they tended to regard these phenomena as essentially transient, trivial and not worthy of investigation. Freud on the other hand emphasised that all behaviour was goal-directed, even though the goals might be hidden (unconscious), and that events of this sort could have a special significance.

In their early studies of hysteria, Breuer and Freud noticed that the peculiar behaviour of their patient made sense in terms of an event from her past that she had apparently forgotten. Her symptom was a re-enactment of the past, and when the memory of the incident which had provoked the symptom was brought into consciousness, that symptom immediately and permanently disappeared (1893, vol II, p 6).[1] This insight quite literally *made sense* of the symptom, which had previously appeared to have a certain random-ness, and it also pointed to the continuity of personality. Most psycho-dynamic theorists, and the Freudians in particular, look for the causes of adult neuroses in the anxieties of childhood and in the progressive sequence of unconscious conflicts and defences against these feelings.

Psycho-analysis is quite explicit about the secondary role of neurotic symptoms. A neurosis may be defined as a psychogenic condition in which the symptoms are the symbolic expression of an *underlying intrapsychic conflict* whose origins lie in the indi-vidual's childhood history (Laplanche and Pontalis 1973). The close resemblance be-tween this psycho-analytic definition and the conventional psychiatric definitions offered in the nosologies DSM 2 and ICD 8 should be apparent, and this testifies to the profound impact that psycho-analysis has had upon psychiatry. The specific points of influence include a distinction between the superficial symptom and the underlying pathological process, an acceptance of the meaning or symbolic significance of the symptoms and of their relationship to an unconscious conflict. In view of the suggestion made in Chap. 2 that psychological medicine would have much to gain by separating the descriptive from the aetiological components of its definitions, it is worth noting that such a suggestion runs counter to the psycho-analytic tradition. Laplanche and Pontalis (ibid) pointed out that the task of trying to define and understand what is meant by the concept of neurosis tends to become indistinguishable from the psycho-analytic theory itself.

Many behaviour therapists have equated the neurotic disorder with the behavioural symptomatology. Eysenck (1959), for instance, stated that 'there is no neurosis underly-ing the symptom, but merely the symptom itself'. To the analyst, on the other hand, the neurosis cannot be equated with symptomatology. A person may be neurotic but show none of the symptoms of phobia, depression, hysteria and so on. The personality disturb-ances underlying the disorder are the crucial feature of neurosis, and in contrast to the views expressed by behaviour therapists, psycho-analysis suggests that 'the cure of a symptom does not necessarily mean the cure of a neurosis' (Horney 1937). Neurotic symptoms are like the eruptions from a volcano, while the pathogenic conflict, like the volcano, is hidden deep within the individual.

6.2 Repression and the Unconscious

The idea of unconscious mental processes is absolutely central to the psycho-analytic view of psychology. Indeed, it is this emphasis upon the role of unconscious mental processes as determinants of behaviour, as much as any other single factor, that distin-guishes psycho-analysis from other psychological theories.

---

1 References to the Standard Edition of Freud's Complete Psychological Works are given in this form – date of original publication, and volume and page numbers of the Standard Edition.

The term 'unconscious' can be used in several different ways. In its least problematic sense it can be used descriptively to refer to the contents of the mind that are not present in the field of consciousness at any given moment. Its other usages are more important; the unconscious is also a topographical (see below) and a dynamic concept, which was derived from Freud's clinical work. He became convinced that the mind could not be equated with consciousness. There seemed to be contents and forces which, although unconscious, remained active in their effects, and which had a particular significance in the determination of neurotic symptoms.

Breuer and Freud, for instance, pointed to the persistence of early memories; though these memories appeared not to persist at a conscious level, nonetheless they had a powerful effect upon the individual's behaviour and determined the symptomatic expression of neurotic disorder – in this case hysteria (1893, vol II). It is an essential feature of neurotic symptoms that the individual has the experience of something strange and unintelligible happening to him. It may that he has involuntary movements or strange changes in his bodily functions and sensations, as in hysteria; or an overwhelming and inexplicable change of mood, as in the depressive disorders; or the need to act and think in a bizarre manner, as in the case of the obsessional and compulsive disorders. In each of these cases the symptoms appear to break into the personality from some unknown or unconscious source.

Ramsay's (1975) complaints about the comparative lack of attention that behaviour therapists have devoted to the question of the patient's willingness to accept the requirements of the treatment regime (see Chap. 5) stand in contrast to the work of the analysts for whom the concept of resistance is of crucial importance. In the *Introductory Lectures,* Freud describes the significance that this aspect of the patient's behaviour had upon his own ideas. 'The patient, who is suffering so much from his symptoms . . . who is ready to undertake so many sacrifices in time, money, effort and self discipline . . . this same patient puts up a struggle in the interest of his illness against the person who is helping him. How improbable such an assertion must sound' (1917, vol XVI, pp 286–287). Freud regarded this resistance to treatment as a manifestation of the same forces that kept the pathogenic ideas out of the patient's conscious awareness, and the concept of resistance was recognised by Freud as one of the corner-stones of psycho-analysis. It has particular importance in treatment, and the analyst usually aims to overcome the resistance by interpretation. This is 'the ultimate and decisive instrument' in psycho-analysis; all other interventions are of subsidiary importance (Greenson 1967). The interpretation is specifically intended to make the patient conscious of the meaning of an unconscious psychic event.

After his collaboration with Breuer using hypnotism, Freud became increasingly dissatisfied with his results. It occured to him that although hypnosis made a certain amount of material available for the analysis, it kept the resistance hidden from the therapist and therefore established an impenetrable barrier beyond which the analyst could not go. Freud was so impressed by this that he dated the beginning of 'psycho-analysis proper' to the time at which he dispensed with the use of hypnosis.

The resistance was seen as evidence of powerful underlying forces which opposed any alteration in the patient's condition, the same forces, in fact, which caused the condition (1917, vol XVI, p 293). There is therefore a close link between the concepts of resistance, repression and the unconscious, and Freud suggested that the concept of the unconscious was itself derived from the theory of repression (1923, vol XIX, p 15). An idea or memory may, because it is unacceptable to the ego for some reason, become repressed; it remains within the mind – outside conscious awareness, but still operative, and under certain circumstances it may re-emerge into consciousness. Repression is the purposeful exclusion from consciousness of wishes, ideas or impulses which are unacceptable to the ego; generally these are of a sexual or aggressive nature. In this sense, repression may be regarded as a specific defence mechanism, and it is one that is especially common in conversion hysteria.

In his refusal to equate the mind with the world of conscious experience, Freud was to a large extent following the tradition established by others in Germany. Herbart, Leibniz, Helmholtz and Fechner had each worked with the idea of the unconscious, but it was for Freud to develop a systematic account of the operation of unconscious forces and to apply this to the neuroses. He wrote of hysteria that the patient's mind was 'full of active yet unconscious ideas; all . . . symptoms proceed from such ideas. It is in fact the most striking character of the hysterical mind to be ruled by them' (1912, vol XII, p 262). The unconscious impulses were not below the threshold of consciousness because they lacked sufficient intensity to maintain themselves in the conscious mind; indeed, in Freud's view the opposite was often the case. It was the unconscious needs and impulses that were frequently the most potent psychological determinants; these remained unconscious only because they were actively excluded from consciousness.

The concept of defence appeared very early in Freud's writings, but for a middle period of almost 30 years it was replaced by the similar notion of repression. In his later work he returned to the notion of defence, and in *The Problem of Anxiety* (1936) he developed the idea that far from being the result of repression, anxiety was the *cause* of repression.

6.3 The Structure of the Mind

In Freudian theory, the structure or topography of the mind includes a number of specific subsystems, each of which has different functions and characteristics. In the *New Introductory Lectures,* Freud referred to this as 'the anatomy of the mental personality'. In the earlier of his two topographical systems, Freud distinguished between the Conscious, Pre-conscious and Unconscious systems: he was later to reject this formulation. In *The Ego and The Id* (1923), Freud proposed a new personality structure, in which the three subsystems of Id, Ego and Super-ego comprised the whole personality.

The id *(das Es)* is the instictive part of the personality; its contents are unconscious and it is generally represented as a reservoir of instinctual energy or drive-force.[2] It includes the sexual instincts, the somatic origins of which can be traced to the oral, anal and genital zones of the body, and it also includes the aggressive instinct. Freud insisted that the instinctual drives were based upon the bodily structure of the organism and rejected the idea of occasional, transitory human instincts, which were so popular at the time (cf. William James and William McDougall). At first, Freud would tolerate no dissent from his thesis that the conflict underlying neurotic disorders was centred upon sexuality. Largely as a result of Adler's ideas, he later admitted that non-sexual factors might lead

---

2 Although it is often translated as 'instinct', the word *'Trieb'* carries the implications of irresistible pressure rather than simply of direction to a predetermined goal. The Freudian concept of *Trieb* implies pressure that is relatively indeterminate and is usually better translated as 'drive'.

to an unconscious conflict. His notion of an aggressive and destructive instinct *(Thanatos)* was an attempt to incorporate a non-sexual instinct into his theory, though the inclusion of aggression as one of the basic Freudian drives runs into some difficulties because of its lack of any clear somatic foundation. For this reason it remains the subject of considerable controversy, and even Fenischel, otherwise one of the most loyal and orthodox Freudians, found the Thanatos notion confused and implausible. Melanie Klein, on the other hand, gave a central position to aggression in her own theory and attributed to it many of the properties that Freud reserved for the libido.

The id is primitive and disorganised; it presses for release of its instinctual tension according to the Pleasure Principle, and these needs and drives press for immediate gratification. The ego is similar to what each of us means when he refers to the 'self': it compromises those aspects of the personality which are responsible for perceiving, understanding, reasoning, feeling and choosing (Hendrick 1958). Whereas the id includes those mental attributes formerly ascribed to the System Unconscious, the ego incorporates the attributes which were previously included in the System Conscious. 'The ego represents what may be called reason and commonsense, in contrast to the id, which contains the passions' (1923, vol XIX, p 25); Freud also used the metaphor of a horse and its rider for the id and ego. The ego is absent in the infant and is an achievement of maturation in the adult: Freud described it as a 'precipitate' of the experiences of the individual in his encounters with the external world. It is the ego that develops the role of reality testing, and as the id serves the Pleasure Principle, so the ego serves the Reality Principle. The functions of the ego are partly synthetic insofar as they operate to maintain the organism as a whole and to reconcile the primitive demands of the id and the moral mandates of the super-ego.

The third agency, the super-ego, is a specialised part of the ego. Its nearest equivalent in common language is the conscience, though Freud's concept of the super-ego differs from this in several important ways. Most importantly, Freud recognised that censorship of the super-ego could be unconscious. The obsessional neurotic 'behaves as if he were dominated by a sense of guilt, of which, however, he knows nothing, so that we must call it an unconscious sense of guilt, in spite of the apparent contradiction in terms' (1907, vol IX, p 123).

In Freudian theory, the super-ego is based on the resolution of the Oedipus complex when the child stops trying to satisfy his Oedipal wishes and internalises the parental prohibitions. It is at this point that Freud suggests that a fundamental difference between the sexes occurs. In the boy, the Oedipus complex and the threat of castration are closely interwoven, and the super-ego is built upon their resolution. For girls it is suggested that the castration complex prepares for the Oedipus complex instead of destroying it, and that the complex is not resolved until comparatively late, and then only incompletely.[3] At a later stage, the super-ego is refined by exposure to other social and cultural factors – education, religion, morality and so forth, but it remains essentially an internalisation of the parental prohibitions. Freud also explicitly stated that the super-ego is not based upon an identification with the parents themselves but upon an identification with the parental *agency* – that is, with the parents' super-ego (1933, vol XXII, p 64).

---

3 In Freud's view, women acquired a less effective super-ego than men (1933, vol XXII, p 129).

6.4 Regression and Infantile Sexuality

Much of the early criticism of Freud's ideas was fuelled by moral indignation. It was thought that his views were irreligious and amoral, and his demonstration of the sexual impulses of children was especially shocking to many. Shortly after the publication of the *Studies in Hysteria,* Breuer withdrew from his collaboration with Freud, and one of the principal reasons for this was probably their disagreement over the significance of sexuality in the causation of neuroses.

In his clinical practice, Freud consistently found that infantile sexual impulses persisted in an unconscious but active form and exerted a powerful effect upon the adult neuroses. He showed that the unconscious sexual wishes of the adult which gave rise to the psychoneurotic disorders were directly related to the infantile period of development during the first 5 years of life. The significance of this period is that it constitutes the foundations of adult sexuality, and that every adult who is frustrated or thwarted in his sexual behaviour regresses to a more primitive stage of sexual functioning in order to gain satisfaction. Freud described the neurotic as quite literally living in the past (1917, vol XVI, p 365). The neurotic symptoms provide a substitute satisfaction for the individual who is faced by frustration; they permit a regression of the libido to earlier and happier times when the libido was able to gain satisfaction. The symptom or symptom-complex repeats this earlier infantile kind of satisfaction, distorted by the censorship arising from the present conflict and mingled with ailments from the precipitating causes of the disorder.

The libido is a biological concept used to refer to the energy of the sexual instinct – the driving force of the personality. In his *Collected Papers* (1924), Freud spoke of it in electro-dynamic or hydro-dynamic terms and described it as being like 'a fluid electrical current', 'something which is capable of increase, decrease, displacement or discharge'. This energy is channelled and directed during the innate, biologically-determined phases of childhood development. Karl Abraham, one of Freud's chief disciples, developed the libido theory in a series of papers, and it was Abraham's work that most influenced Freud's thinking in this area; as a result of his researches, Freud came to regard libidinal energy as organised differently during the different stages of infantile development. In the first phase, the oral phase, the libido is bound mainly to the mouth, and the sources of pleasure for the infant are his own body and the breast that feeds him. Because of the inability to differentiate internal and external sources of stimulation, even the mother's breast is conceived of as belonging to the ego.

During the second developmental stage, which occurs approximately between the ages of 2 and 4, Freud suggested that the focus of libidinal interest begins to shift from the oral to the anal region, and the infant's pleasures become associated with the retention and expulsion of faeces. Unlike the comparatively passive oral phase, the anal phase is directed towards the external world and relates to the parents in terms of defiance, submission and feelings of power. It is at this time that the symbolic significance of giving and withholding is established.

In the third, phallic phase of libidinal development, the libidinal gratifications of both sexes become centred upon the genital organs, and it is at about this time that the little girl begins to develop feelings of 'penis-envy'.

It is during the phallic phase that the Oedipus complex occurs. This plays a basic role in the individual's personality development: indeed the neurotic's failure to resolve the Oedipus complex (in which the libido is attached to the image of the parent figures) forms the nucleus of the psycho-neuroses (1925, vol XX, p 55). For the boy the resolution of his Oedipal feelings is connected with the fear of castration: for girls, Freud suggested a different biologically-determined course of development. The girl is resentful of her lack of a penis; but at the same time, because of this, she is not affected by fears of castration and is likely to spend a longer period in the Oedipal phase.

These phases of infantile sexual development are followed by a latency period, which persists until increased levels of libido at puberty revive sexual interests. It is during the latency period that there is an intensification of repression leading to an amnesia of the earlier years. After puberty, the boy maintains his penis-interest and continues along the same developmental course as before; but the girl must now become aware of her vagina, and therefore, Freud suggested, of her feminine and passive role, and must renounce her interest in the clitoris.

These various phases overlap and interact in the course of development, and it is important to note that no phase is entirely given up. Freud presents the analogy of an advancing army which leaves garrisons on its route to send forward supplies and to provide a line of retreat in the event of being checked and driven back. The tendency of the forces to occupy and fortify one of the earlier positions is called fixation: the retreat of the force to this point under adverse circumstances is the process of regression. The neurotic disorder is prompted by the current difficulties in the patient's adult environment, but the disorder itself reflects the regression. 'The aetiology of the (neuroses) . . . is to be looked for in the individual's developmental history . . . neuroses are acquired only in early childhood . . . even though their symptoms may not make their appearance until much later' (1938, vol XXIII, pp 156 and 185). In this, the neurotic disorder is a form of repetition. In an earlier work, Freud had described hysterics as suffering mainly from their reminiscences, but he later modified his views on this, since the repetition of the neurotic, far from being synonymous with memory, is actually an alternative to, and a substitute for, reminiscence. The neurotic repeats instead of remembering (1914, vol XII, p 151).

6.5 The Actual Neuroses

Freud made a clear distinction between the actual neuroses and the psycho-neuroses. The former were a comparatively simple form of neurosis, the direct result of incomplete sexual satisfaction, whereas the psycho-neuroses were more complicated and were caused by a conflict between the ego and the sexual instincts. The term 'actual neurosis' first appeared in Freud's writings in 1898 to denote anxiety neurosis and neurasthenia, though he was later to include various psychosomatic and hypochondriacal disorders within this category.

The actual neuroses differ from the psycho-neuroses in several respects. In the first place the actual neuroses are *not* caused by unresolved infantile conflicts, but have their origins in the subject's present circumstances: (the adjective 'actual' is used here in the sense of *temporal* actuality). In both types of neurosis the causes are sexual, but in the actual neuroses the mechanism is somatic rather than psychological. 'The neuroses [are] . . . without exception disturbances of the sexual function, the so-called *"actual neuroses"* being the direct toxic expression of such disturbances and the *psycho-neuroses* their mental expression' (1925, vol XX, p 25).

In the case of anxiety neurosis, the cause may be found in the non-discharge of sexual excitation which results in 'a deflection of somatic sexual excitation . . . and the consequent abnormal employment of that excitation' (1895, vol III, p 108), and in neurasthenia, in some sort of incomplete sexual satisfaction such as masturbation or spontaneous emission. This differs from the earlier account of neurasthenia given by Beard, in which sexual factors were only one of many determinants. The symptoms of the actual neuroses also differ from those of the psycho-neurotic disorders in that they are *a direct outcome of the absence or inadequacy of sexual satisfaction,* rather than a symbolic expression of some intrapsychic conflict.

The theoretical significance of this distinction is that the actual neuroses cannot be treated by psycho-analysis, because their symptoms lack any symbolic meaning that can be brought into the patient's consciousness. Freud maintained that these disorders were to be explained in neuro-chemical rather than psychological terms. 'I cannot regard the genesis of the symptoms (of the actual neuroses) . . . as anything but toxic' (1912, vol XII, p 248).

Freud appears to have accepted that 'abnormal' sexual practices had a biological significance independent of cultural definitions and that they had a *direct* and straightforward causal influence upon the actual neuroses. He described how manual masturbation led to one sort of actual neurosis, whereas another form of actual neurosis would immediately appear in place of the first if the patient changed to some other form of abnormal and incomplete sexual behaviour (1917, vol XVI, p 386). Nonetheless, the symptom of an actual neurosis can be the first stage of a psycho-neurotic symptom. Freud suggested that although the pure cases of anxiety neurosis were usually the most marked, the symptoms of anxiety more often occurred at the same time as symptoms of neurasthenia, hysteria or depression, and in his earlier writings he often used the term 'mixed neurosis' to refer to the combination of different types of neurosis. Mixed neurosis implied not merely a complicated mixture of the two sorts of neurotic symptomatology, but also 'the admixture of several specific aetiologies' (1895, vol III, p 113).

Freud's explanation of the actual neuroses was entirely consistent with his libido theory. The libidinal energy was directed towards its release in orgasm and if deprived of this satisfaction, the energy remained in the system pressing for discharge. In this way it became converted into anxiety. Although anxiety is now regarded as a central concept in understanding neurosis, this is a comparatively recent development. Prior to the 1920s anxiety was regarded as of only incidental importance, and in his early work Freud consigned anxiety to the category of actual neuroses and explained it as a direct physiological reaction to sexual frustration. He never entirely abandoned this position, but in *The Problem of Anxiety* he introduced an entirely different account of anxiety, in which it was seen as a signal of some internal, intrapsychic threat. In this second formulation, the neurosis developed as an attempt to cope with anxiety.

Freud's interest in the actual neuroses was somewhat eclipsed by his later concentration upon the psycho-neuroses, and since few other analysts have shown much interest in this topic it has been rather overlooked. Nonetheless, in a retrospective look at his formulation of the actual neuroses, Freud suggested that although his ideas might have been only a rough outline of a complicated subject, they remained fundamentally sound (1925, vol XX, p 26).

6.6 The Psycho-neuroses

The concept of psycho-neurosis appears very early in Freud's writings. *In The Neuro-psychoses of Defence* (1894, vol III) he presented a psychological theory of phobias, obsessions and conversion hysteria. The theory of repression (or defence) first appeared in this paper, and Freud was to describe this as the 'cornerstone on which the whole structure of psychoanalysis rests. It is the most essential part of it' (1914, vol XIV, p 16).

Freud divided the psycho-neuroses into two categories, the transference neuroses (phobias, obsessions and conversion hysteria), in which the patient responds to frustration by investing libido in fantasised objects, and the narcissistic neuroses. Table 3 shows the Freudian concepts of neurosis in relation to current psychiatric usage. Of course, it is not possible to achieve a precise matching, both because of historical changes in the meanings of the concepts themselves and because of the ambiguities which are inherent in both systems. The Freudian distinction between the actual neuroses and the psycho-neuroses is one that is not made in the psychiatric nosologies, and the concept of psycho-neurosis strays beyond the conventional limits of 'neurosis' into that of 'psychosis'. The concept of narcissistic neurosis has also disappeared from present-day usage. Freud used it to refer to those cases in which the libido had been withdrawn from the outside world and redirected towards the ego itself. Initially, the term had been used by Freud in an attempt to extend psycho-analytic principles to the psychoses, though he was later to limit its use to certain depressive conditions, and it most nearly corresponds to what psychiatrists would now call manic-depressive psychosis.

Freud used the concept of repression to contrast the psycho-neuroses (more precisely, the transference neuroses) with the actual neuroses. The symptoms of the psycho-neuroses were regarded as a symbolic expression of unresolved infantile conflicts. The conflict is caused by frustration which deprives the libido of satisfaction, causing it to seek new sources of release in regression. If these regressions arouse no objection from the ego, the libido will achieve some real, though perverse, form of satisfaction – as in the sexual perversions. But despite this important difference, Freud noted that the sexual perversions shared with the neuroses features of regression, fixation and repression, and suggested that they too were accessible to treatment by psycho-analysis (1905, vol VII, p 232).

Table 3. The Freudian concepts of neurosis

Freudian concepts	Actual neurosis	Psychoneurosis		
		Transference neuroses	Narcissistic neuroses	
			Narcissistic neuroses	Paraphrenias
Current psychiatric usage	Anxiety neurosis, hypochondriacal neurosis, neurasthenia	Obsessional-compulsive, phobic and hysterical neuroses	Manic-depressive psychosis	Paranoid schizophrenia

It is an essential feature of the *neurotic* conflict, on the other hand, that the new objects and paths to libidinal satisfaction should be unacceptable to the ego, which opposes the new attempt to gain satisfaction. 'One part of the personality champions certain wishes while another part opposes them and fends them off. Without such a conflict there is no neurosis' (1917, vol XVI, p 349). The frustrated libidinal impulses must seek some indirect way of finding a new form of satisfaction, and this results in the formation of neurotic symptoms. In all cases the pathogenic conflict is between the ego and sexuality, and the ego actively initiates defensive processes in response to the danger. This frequently takes the form of repression, though the ego may also use other defence mechanisms to protect itself from conscious awareness of unacceptable impulses: these include projection, reaction formation, denial, displacement, undoing and rationalisation. In each of these cases, the neurotic remains in a state of basic conflict, since he must keep himself unconscious of the defences that he is using and of the true significance of the unacceptable elements. Because of this, repression has a paradigmatic importance in Freudian theory, and Freud referred to the other defences as 'surrogates of repression' (1926, vol XX, p 119).

6.7 Little Hans

In his writings, Freud made considerable use of his own clinical material, both as evidence of the practical effectiveness of psycho-analysis and as illustrative material for its theoretical principles. One of the best-known cases was that of Little Hans, first published under the title *'Analysis of a Phobia in a Five Year Old Boy'* (1909, vol X, pp 5–149). Although atypical in some ways, the case is significant because it provides the first example of a child analysis. It also confirmed Freud's views about the sexuality of childhood and has been used by analysts as a basic substantiation of psycho-analytic theory. In this case Freud was able to 'observe directly' the sexual impulses and wishes that are so deeply hidden in adults.

Little Hans[4] had developed strong fears of being bitten by a horse, which developed after he had seen a horse fall down in the street one day. It is a central task of the analysis to establish the symbolic meaning of the horse. Hans' problem is described in terms of his Oedipal desires for his mother, with whom he was allowed to sleep in his father's absence. Freud suggests that Hans developed a wish that his father should be permanently absent (i.e. be dead) so that Hans could replace him in his mother's bed: because of his love for his father, his Oedipal desires and the death wishes were denied direct expression. Hans' first statement of his phobia and his fear of being bitten represented his fears of castration by his father for his Oedipal longings. The repressed libidinal energy had found release in some new form, showing itself as anxiety.

It is as a means of coping with this anxiety that the symptom arises. The mind erects 'mental barriers in the nature of precautions, inhibitions, or prohibitions; and it is these defensive structures that appear to us in the form of phobias' (1909, vol X, p 117).

---

4 Because of the limitations of space in this chapter, the account of Little Hans is necessarily abbreviated and cannot convey a true impression of Freud's analytic writing. The reader who wishes more than the skeletal outline offered here might refer to the original work: for a critical discussion of this work the reader might consider Wolpe and Rachman (1960).

Neurotic symptoms take the form of a compromise which disguise the original impulse at the same time as allowing it some form of indirect expression. Hans' fear of horses was actually quite complex. Behind his fear of being bitten was a deeper fear of horses falling down. The symbolic meaning of a falling horse is presented by Freud as the father dying, as well as the mother in childbirth. (When Hans was $3^1/_2$ years old, the mother had given birth to a baby sister, and this event also plays a large part in the analysis.) The symptom operates to hide this from Hans by transferring the anxiety from its true, but unacceptable, source to the overt symptom. At the same time the compromise solution that the symptom represents permits some part of his repressed desire to achieve release, for example in his inability to leave the house and therefore to leave his mother.

As a result of bringing to light the repressed complexes, Freud reports that Hans lost his fear of horses and developed a better relationship with his father. Some years later Freud met Hans when he was a young man and he had retained his therapeutic gains and was free from any neurotic problems.

6.8 Neo-freudian Theories

Many critics of psycho-analysis have under-estimated both the complexity of psycho-analytic theory itself, and more particularly, the diversity of psycho-analytic viewpoints. There can be little doubt that in his emphasis upon constitutional and organic determinants, Freud showed a serious neglect of the important role played by social and cultural factors. He frequently mistook cultural for biological-instinctual phenomena, and this was the focus of concern for several of the neo-Freudians. One of the basic issues that divides the schools of psycho-analysis is Freud's libido theory, and particularly the role of infantile sexuality in personality formation and in the determination of adult neuroses. Jung's departure from orthodox Freudian theory was based upon his desire to avoid what he saw as an undue emphasis upon infantile sexuality and the Oedipus Complex. The non-libido theorists (including Horney, Adler, Fromm and Sullivan) also reacted against the biological-drive formulation and emphasised the self and its social and interpersonal experiences as the crucial determinants of behaviour.

6.8.1 Adler

In 1911, Alfred Adler was the first to break away from Freud's inner circle. His theory of 'Individual Psychology' was based upon the social and interpersonal experiences of the child. Although these factors are also of obvious importance to the Freudian account, they do not occupy the primary role that Adler granted them.

The Individual Psychology account of the neuroses (and of human behaviour in general) is based upon two main principles: (a) inferiority feelings which are the result of man's physical endowments or his social situation and (b) his strivings for mastery, control or power in an attempt to compensate for these feelings. In the case of the neurotic, the attempted compensation is exaggerated and unrealistic, and it leads to the person's becoming self-centred rather than outwardly-directed towards the social and physical world.

In his early studies, Adler investigated the psychological techniques by which individuals learned to cope with 'organ inferiorities' such as bodily defects. A frequently quoted example is that of Demosthenes, who became a great orator in compensation for a childhood speech defect: other stutterers might use the same defect as an excuse to defend their self-esteem against the threat of failure. Similarly, every normal child starts life from a position of helplessness, then strives increasingly to control his sense of inferiority before the environment. The point at which the individual feels most inferior is determined by specific organ inferiorities, and by social and interpersonal factors. It is precisely at this point of weakness that the compensatory strivings for superiority are most marked (Adler 1946). The drive towards power, prestige, superiority or perfection plays a central part in Adler's theory, and the style of life by which the child learns to cope with his feelings carries through to adulthood.

Like Freud, Adler recognised the first 5 years of life as crucial for personality structure, but he believed that human behaviour was to be explained in terms of *present* ambitions, hopes and strivings towards the future, rather than by biological drives or the unconscious imprint of past experiences. Adler was unimpressed by the Freudian concepts of the unconscious and repression. Although the patient might be unaware of their inner life, this was not due to repressions, unconscious processes or resistances. This denial of basic Freudian concepts led many analysts to regard Adler's system not as false, but as superficial, dealing with the secondary gains of neurosis rather than the primary causes (Hendrick 1958).

In the neurotic, the individual's goals are unreal and egocentric, and are primarily an attempt to attract the attention of other people. 'The entire picture of the neurosis as well as all its symptoms are influenced by, nay, even wholly provoked by an imaginary fictitious goal' (Adler 1918); this goal is the universal drive to power, which is unusually marked in the neurotic. The neurotic shows 'no single trait which cannot likewise be demonstrated in the healthy individual' (ibid), although the neurotic character is incapable of adjusting to reality because it is focused upon an impossible and fictitious goal.

Adler introduced the concepts of 'sibling rivalry' and 'inferiority complex', and the accessibility of these notions to people outside psycho-analysis led to their rapid and widespread acceptance. Indeed, they have now passed into common usage. But despite its initial widespread acceptance at the time, Adler's Individual Psychology as a system is now practically extinct, although his ideas had a marked influence upon Karen Horney's work.

6.8.2 Horney

Karen Horney was also one of Freud's faithful disciples, but after emigrating to New York she made a radical break with him. Her definition of psycho-analysis as 'certain basic trends of thought concerning the role of unconscious processes and the ways in which they find expression, and . . . a form of therapeutic treatment that brings these processes to awareness' (Horney 1937), although rather general, is fairly orthodox; but like Adler's theory, which had a marked influence on her work, Horney rejected the libido theory and the structural approach (id, ego, superego). Unlike Adler, for whom anxiety was a comparatively minor concept, Horney gave a central role to anxiety in her theory. It is anxiety and the individual's attempts to defend himself against feelings of anxiety that lie at the heart of the neurotic disorders, and for Horney, an investigation into the causes of anxiety was an investigation into the causes of the neuroses.

One of the basic causes of anxiety was 'inevitably a lack of genuine warmth and affection in childhood' (Horney 1937). Coupled with the fundamental helplessness of the child, this leads to hostility, which in turn creates anxiety, since the child is unable to give free expression to these hostile feelings. Horney refers to this attitude as 'the basic anxiety; it is inseparably interwoven with a basic hostility' (ibid), and it is from these two opposing forces that the neurotic conflict arises. The simultaneous need to approach others and to avoid or to oppose them, leads to the neurotic attitudes of submissiveness, withdrawal or aggressiveness. Because of her approach, she was comparatively uninterested in specific symptoms and in the underlying personality determinants of the neurotic behaviour. Instead, she attaches absolute importance to the interpersonal and cultural situations in which the neurosis finds expression (Wyss 1966).

She recognised that psycho-analysis as a sytem has always been in danger of stagnation through deference to Freud's own achievements. Horney stressed the cultural implications of the concept of neurosis. What might be considered abnormal in our own culture, or in our own time, might be regarded as appropriate in other times and places. Both Fromm and Horney pointed out how Freud's ideas were restricted by his own cultural background. Fromm (1960) wrote that 'Freud was so imbued with the spirit of his culture that he could not go beyond certain limits which were set by it. These very limits became limitations for his understanding . . . of the sick individual . . . of the normal individual . . . of the irrational phenomena operating in social life.' Horney (1936) was concerned with the possibility that neuroses may be moulded by socio-cultural processes 'in essentially the same way as 'normal' character formation', and that the neurotic conflict was not simply one of coping with instinctual intrapsychic drives, but one of adapting to the conflicting demands that society imposes upon its members.

Freud's conclusion that women are more jealous than men was based upon his view that the anatomical differences between the sexes inevitably leads girls to be envious of boys. This penis envy is later translated into an envy of other women's relationships with men (i. e. their possession of other men). Other analysts have given even more emphasis to this anatomically-based penis envy in women. Helen Deutsch, for instance, believed that the psychology of women is primarily determined by their attempts to compensate for their anatomical defect (Deutsch 1944).

Horney, however, has always been one of the most articulate critics of this aspect of Freudian theory. She concluded that there were no basic psychological differences between the sexes, and insofar as penis envy exists, it is not biologically-, but culturally-determined, and is more likely to represent an envy of the masculine social advantages than an envy of his anatomical advantages. Freud's views on this matter represented an over-generalisation from a culturally limited viewpoint. She cited anthropological evidence of the wide variations in the expression of jealousy by men and women that exist in different societies, and suggested that Freud's pronouncements about the specific guilts, competitiveness, sibling rivalry, etc. were based upon a restricted view of human nature. The Freudian over-valuation of biological determinants to the neglect of cultural factors was one of the greatest defects in his work. 'Freud's disregard of cultural factors not only leads to false generalisations, but to a large extent blocks an understanding of the real forces which motivate our attitudes and actions' (Horney 1937).

All analysts, including Freud, accept that repressed hostility is a frequent cause of anxiety. But whereas Freud explains this in terms of his instinct theory, Horney sees the hostility in terms of the individual's experiences with his socio-cultural environment. In her own formulation, the essence of the neurotic condition is *basic anxiety,* by which is meant 'the feeling (originating in childhood) of being isolated and helpless in a potentially hostile world' (Horney 1946). It is the pattern of responses by which the person learns to cope with this culturally-determined basic anxiety (Horney refers to these as safety devices) that constitutes the symptoms of the neurotic disorder.

The ego protects itself against basic anxiety by erecting defences, and in Horney's view, these neurotic defences themselves can cause further anxiety, since they may be in conflict with each other. Thompson (1950) illustrates this by the case of a child who has developed powerful needs for success and recognition, but later experience leads him to despise and devalue such needs. This produces the conflict between secret ambitions and the need to appear outwardly modest and inconspicuous, and as a result of this conflict the person becomes an under-achiever, unable to assert himself. This is intolerable to the ambitious part of his personality, and as a result he must either experience an increase in anxiety or add new defences against that anxiety, such as the belief that others are obstructing his progress.

6.8.3 Fromm

Like Horney, Erich Fromm was opposed to the biological emphasis of Freud's work: as with all psycho-analysts, Fromm looks to the child's experiences within the family as the crucial determinants of personality development, but whereas Horney substituted an alternative socio-cultural account of the determination of drives, Fromm criticised Freud's theory of drives from a different perspective. Unlike Horney, whose explanation of neurosis relies upon the notion of basic anxiety, Fromm argued that there is a fundamental and crucial distinction between the biological drives of animals and the human drives. Whereas animal drives are predetermined and limited in their operation, human behaviour is flexible. Man is, in principle, free to choose whether or not he will obey his drives, and Fromm's basic premise is that of individuation, man's attempt to achieve self-realisation and freedom from his biological nature. This freedom from biological restraint imposes its own demands upon all individuals. Individuation is not an easy process, and it is man's freedom from his biological nature that permits the formation of neurosis. For the neurotic, the threat of freedom proves intolerable. In the tension between the impulse towards free individuation and the security of primary (infantile) emotional ties, the neurotic opts for security rather than freedom: in his attempts to avoid feelings of isolation and loneliness the neurotic uses mechanisms of escape. These neurotic solutions take various forms. The person may, for instance, adopt a pattern of blind conformity to cultural expectations (automaton conformity), and much of Fromm's work is concerned with the issue of conformity and authoritarianism (e. g. *Fear of Freedom* 1960). But these neurotic attempts to solve the problem of isolation must fail because man cannot reunite himself with the world in the way that was possible before the development of individuality.

Fromm's theory suffers from a number of drawbacks, not the least of which is its somewhat vague and 'philosophical' style. Another problem with his account of neurosis (as with those of Adler and Horney) is that although it introduces social factors into the discussion, it reduces their psychological significance to an over-simplified form. The phenomena of neurosis are too complex and varied to be easily explained solely in terms of such concepts as the need for mastery, basic anxiety or fear of individuation. This weakness of the neo-Freudian theories of neurosis is linked to their neglect of the specific symptoms of the neurotic disorders. These neo-Freudian accounts focus upon character neurosis, a term which is widely used, but has no exact meaning. This approach transcends the distinction between neuroses with symptoms and those without symptoms by its overall emphasis upon personality organisation, but degrades the importance of symptoms in the pursuit of intrapsychic events. Admittedly, the clinical investigation of neurosis was not one of Fromm's principal aims, but Adler and Horney also neglect this problem of symptoms and attempt to conceptualise and explain neurosis in general terms of personality adjustment.

6.9 The Evaluation of Psycho-analysis

On the fundamentally important question of 'evidence', there is good reason to believe that many psycho-analysts, and Freud in particular, hold a mistaken view of their own role. Freud wrote of his critics that 'the main obstacle to agreement lay in the fact that my opponents regarded psycho-analysis as a product of my speculative imagination and were unwilling to believe in the long, patient and *unbiased*[5] work which had gone into its making' (1925, vol XX, p 50).

The first objection to this view that the analyst's clinical observations could be unbiased is a general one. Perceptions occur in a framework of beliefs, expectations, values and so forth: the analyst's perceptions of the patient are not veridical and unbiased in the way that Freud assumed. Beyond this, the complexity of the patient-doctor interaction is underestimated. Truax (1966) found that even the supposedly non-directive interviews of Rogers contained their own implicit reinforcements and directives, of which the therapist was unaware. Whether he likes it or not, the therapist influences the patient's responses.

Freud was also ambivalent about the analyst's role in treatment. Contrary to his own directive that the analyst should be 'impenetrable to the patient' and 'like a mirror', Freud also stated that 'during the analysis [the patient] had to be told many things that he could not say himself, that he had to be presented with thoughts which he had so far shown no signs of possessing, and that his attention had to be turned in the direction from which his father was expecting something to come' (1909, vol X, p 104). Elsewhere he stated that he would 'stand obstinately by my suspicions till I had overcome the patients' disingenuousness and compelled them to confirm my views' (1917, vol XVI, p 386). The analysis therefore has many of the characteristics of education or indoctrination, in which the structure of psycho-analysis is imposed upon the patient. This leads to further difficulties associated with the process of interpretation, to which analysts attach so much weight as a special sort of evidence. The patient's acceptance of the interpretation provides no evidence that the interpretation itself was an accurate or 'true' identification of unconscious material. Farrell (1967) characterised the process of interpretation as principally a means of transforming the patient into a 'Freudian-type' of person. In short, the analyst is likely to discover whatever he looks for.

The uncertainties surrounding the psycho-analyst's use of clinical observation and interpretation render them a poor vehicle for gathering evidence about the validity of psycho-analytic theory. Freud was mistaken in his view that his theory was supported by such a 'wealth of reliable observations . . . [that it was] independent of experimental verification' (Freud's comments to Rosenzweig, cited in Postman 1962). There are,

---

5 My italics.

however, many problems inherent in any attempt to put Freud's theoretical statements to the test. Farrell (1951, 1961) stated that 'psycho-analytic theory is *qua* theory, unbelievably bad', and that certain aspects of the theory are untestable.

Karl Popper's dissatisfaction with the psycho-analytic theories of Freud and Adler was rooted in the apparent paradox that their explanatory power was *too great*. The theories were able to explain practically everything that happened, and conversely, whatever happened seemed to verify the theory. It is certainly true that Freud and most of his colleagues believed that psycho-analytic theory was constantly being verified by their clinical observations, and in one sense there are no eventualities that could contradict them. This is their greatest flaw: they are not falsifiable.

Popper (1963) presented the criterion of testability or falsifiability, as a means of distinguishing between the statements of the empirical sciences and those of pseudo-science. Another expression of this is that a scientific theory must be capable of learning from its mistakes. Those propositions which we cannot (in principle) put to the test and *disconfirm* belong to the realm of religion or mythology. At the same time this criterion of falsifiability must not be confused with the issue of meaningfulness or of truth: because a statement is untestable does not mean that it is necessarily nonsensical or untrue.

This view of science has been important and influential, and although there are philosophical problems inherent in this position (cf. Kuhn 1970), it is generally agreed that theoretical propositions should be amenable to some sort of stringent test. Harzen and Miles (1961) argued that this demand for evidence, although difficult to state in a way which is itself free from theoretical objections, remains valid. The problem that psycho-analysis must then face in one form or another is this – what could count as satisfactory evidence for rejecting particular aspects of the theory?

The Pleasure Principle, for instance, is crucial to Freudian theory (repression and unconscious processes depend upon it), yet there is no way of putting it to the test. The reduction of tension within the psychic system is a vague notion which escapes empirical scrutiny, because there is no indication of what form this tension takes, or how it might be measured. The nearest principles from experimental psychology, the drive-reduction hypothesis and the Law of Effect, have themselves been rejected because they are either tautologous or incorrect (Eysenck 1976). Another illustration of the tendency of psycho-analytical theory to distance itself from the possibility of empirical investigation can be found in Freud's statements about the distribution of libido. 'All through the subject's life his ego remains the great reservoir of his libido, from which object-cathexes are sent out and into which libido can stream back again from the objects' (1925, vol XX, p 56). It is not clear what criteria we could adopt to test the truth or accuracy of such a statement.

Similarly, psycho-analysis proposes that obsessional-neurosis and anal-eroticism are related, in the sense that obsessional traits are defence mechanisms against anal-eroticism that has been repressed in early childhood by over-zealous toilet training. Kline (1968) made an empirical study of this issue using four questionnaire measures of obsessionality and the Blacky Pictures projective test. His results showed a significant positive correlation between obsessionality as measured on three of the objective tests and the measures of anality on the projective test. Kline suggests that his findings broadly support the Freudian theory. Yet in the same paper he notes that the Freudian theory links anality to fixation at the retentive stage, and that 'perhaps, there should be a negative correlation with the [anal] expulsive score'. His own results show four *positive* correlations, one of which was statistically significant. Because of this vagueness of the theory, it is frequently difficult (as in this case) to know whether or not results confirm its predictions or not.

The same state of affairs can be found in many other areas of the psycho-analytic theory of neurosis. Either the theory itself is untestable, or its predictions are equivocal. Stein and Ottenberg (1958) attempted to test the hypothesis that asthmatic attacks represent a psychosomatic defence against smells which would activate unresolved childhood conflicts. The authors claim that their results support the Freudian theory because dirty and unpleasant (anal) smells are more likely to induce attacks than pleasant smells. But despite the authors' conclusions, the most common *single* cause of asthmatic attacks was perfume (ten subjects). This contrasts with only two subjects who mentioned the smell of faeces as a precipitant. One might also take issue with the inclusion of paint, horses and smoke in the category of 'unclean' smells. The results are further weakened by the authors' failure to consider alternative explanations. The asthma may, for instance, be a result of hypersensitivity to certain chemicals, which causes the restriction of air passages to avoid taking in substances to which the person is allergic. Yet again one is faced by the problem that the theory does not specify precisely enough under what conditions the psychosomatic reaction should occur.

The term 'psycho-analysis' has two quite distinct meanings – Freud referred to it as a science of unconscious mental processes, and as a particular method of treating psychological disorders. In its second sense Freud argued that psycho-analysis is a more effective treatment for the psycho-neuroses (hysteria, phobias and the obsessional states) than any other method of treatment (1926, vol XX, p 264).

In trying to evaluate the effectiveness of psycho-analytic treatment, the sheer length of the course of treatment presents one of the first difficulties. Heilbrunn (1963) presented the results of his own treatment of patients over a *15-year* period and concluded that only 38% of the patient who had been seen for between 301 and 1350 sessions showed improvement. Other studies have cited higher rates of improvement, but only after selecting out the patients who terminated their treatment prematurely (e. g. Knight 1941): this sort of data manipulation is obviously suspect.

In the evaluation of the effectiveness of psycho-analysis, most authors have neglected the phenomenon of spontaneous recovery. Denker (1946) and Wallace and Whyte (1959) suggested that as many as 70% of neurotics show spontaneous remission of their symptoms without psychotherapy, though this may not be equally true of all the varieties of neurosis. Meyer and Crisp (1970) suggested that obsessional neurosis does not typically show this sort of remission and is often resistant to treatment.

If one accepts the two-thirds spontaneous recovery rate, this leads to some problems for proponents of psycho-analysis, since their own treatment success rates are lower than this. Stuart's (1970) review presented rates of between 24 and 54% improvement for psycho-analytic treatment, and suggested on the basis of these estimates of the rate of spontaneous recovery that psycho-analysis may adversely affect the patient's chances of recovery. This conclusion is probably unwarranted on the basis of any overall estimate of the rate of spontaneous remission for neurosis. Different neuroses appear to show different rates of recovery (Subotnik 1972), and it is not clear that the patients treated by psycho-analysis and those in the spontaneous recovery studies were directly comparable: the processes of patient selection are still inadequately understood. Nonetheless, even the most conservative estimates of spontaneous recovery suggest that between 20% and 40% of neurotics may recover without treatment (Paul 1966; Saslow and Peters 1956), and any evaluation of treatment effectiveness should control for this effect. Few psycho-analytic studies have done so.

A further difficulty is raised by the use of different criteria of improvement in the studies of spontaneous recovery and in psycho-analytic treatment. Because the analytic definition of neurosis goes beyond the symptoms to unconscious personality factors, many psycho-analysts would not accept the simple remission of specific symptoms as evidence of recovery. The *phenotypic* concepts of behaviour therapy, which are concerned with overt behaviour, and the *genotypic* concepts of psycho-analysis, which deal with unobservable psychic forces, are not necessarily independent, but in practice it is often impossible to translate from one system into the other.

It is difficult to reconcile the facts of symptomatic treatment or spontaneous recovery with psycho-analytic theory, since the disappearance of the substitute satisfactions offered by the neurotic symptom should lead to a re-emergence of the libido in some other form of expression. According to Freudian theory, all neurotic symptoms are secondary and superficial. They are symbolic of some unconscious process and are not in themselves the essence of the neurosis. Obsessional ideas, for instance, are *invariably* the expression of transformed self-reproaches originating in some sexual act that was performed with pleasure in childhood and which have re-emerged from repression. In the treatment of neurosis, the analyst aims to make the patient aware of the unconscious meaning of the symptom, and it has been widely assumed that symptomatic treatment of the neuroses is therefore a waste of time. Since the symptom is merely the superficial expression of underlying conflicts and anxieties, the removal of the symptom should leave the basic neurosis unchanged and likely to find some alternative form of expression.

On this issue the analysts and behaviour therapists make quite different predictions. Whereas Freud stated that 'it is impossible to effect the cure of a phobia (and even in certain circumstances dangerous to attempt to do so)' (1909, vol X, p 117) by forcing the patient to confront his phobic stimulus, behaviour therapists have done precisely this. In some cases the exposure has been gradual, as in systematic desensitisation, in others symbolic, as in covert or imaginal sensitisation; in other cases the patient has been faced with in vivo exposure, as in flooding. Each of these symptomatic treatments leads to improvement in phobic disorders without evidence of symptom substitution (Marks 1974). Similarly, obsessional-compulsive disorders improve as a result of enforced ritual-prevention (Levy and Meyer 1971): again, no symptom substitution occurred and there was an additional gain in that the patients experienced less anxiety and depression after the treatment. Mowrer (1976) has described how the direct treatment of enuresis by conditioning methods led to not one single incidence of symptom substitution as predicted by Freudian theory.

Blanchard and Hersen (1976) attempted to explain how psycho-analysts and behaviour therapists have failed to resolve their disagreement over such a fundamental issue as whether or not symptom substitution occurs by suggesting that proponents of each theory have generalised beyond their data. Psycho-analysts, for instance, have been especially interested in hysteria, in which there is an element of secondary gain. This might be expected to lead to symptom substitution (or to relapse) if the treatment consisted merely of symptom removal or symptom supresion. Behaviour therapists, on the other hand, have been more concerned with the phobic, obsessional-compulsive and anxiety disorders. These may be seen as avoidance behaviours which are maintained by the anxiety-reducing properties of the symptomatic behaviours. In such cases, the evidence is much clearer. Symptom substitution in the psycho-analytic sense does not occur.

7. Trait Theories of Neurosis

We cannot understand behaviour simply as a response to the external environment. People seem to act with a degree of consistency in different situations as if they were predisposed towards certain sorts of behaviour. Some people react with anxiety to the slightest threat, whereas others remain free from anxiety under the most stressful conditions. In those people who are psychologically disturbed, it is even more likely that their behaviour will be seen as a result of distinctive individual or personality predispositions. When someone reacts with terror to the sight of a dog, or feels an overwhelming compulsion to wash their hands every time they touch some object in their environment, or believes that they have a fatal illness whenever they have the slightest ache or pain, then it is likely that we will seek to explain their unusual behaviour in personality terms.

This chapter will deal mainly with the personality theories of two psychologists with very different attitudes towards psycho-analysis – Hans Eysenck and Raymond Cattell. Eysenck has consistently and vigorously opposed the formulations of psycho-analysis; Cattell, on the other hand, has been more sympathetic to such views, and many areas of his work reflect the influence of psycho-analysis. Eysenck and Cattell both share a commitment to the validity of a trait-description approach to the neuroses. Unfortunately, it is not at all clear what is to count as a definition of a personality trait, and despite the fact that Allport identified about 18 000 trait names in the English language, there remains considerable disagreement between psychologists as to what is meant by the term. In the most general sense, a trait is a collection of responses bound together by shared characteristics which permit them to be described by a common term. Trait psychology assumes a certain consistency of behaviour across situations, and traits are seen as relatively stable and enduring predispositions acquired through learning, or through constitutional or genetic effects, and which exert fairly generalised effects on behaviour.

Eysenck (1972b) has argued that trait psychology does not provide a *causal* analysis of behaviour, but rather a *descriptive* one; as such it attempts to identify the underlying structures of superficially chaotic and complex forms of behaviour. With respect to the causal and descriptive functions of personality theory, Eysenck could be accused of inviting misunderstanding by the way that his writings tend to switch from the causal to the descriptive level – usually without explicit comment. Cattell, on the other hand, does allow a causal role to trait factors, though he also regards the descriptive function of trait theory as important, arguing that psychologists have paid far too little attention to the basic conceptual foundations upon which their discipline is based. As a result of this neglect, research psychologists are inclined 'to resemble a mob rather than a disciplined army, preferring the looting of more or less immediately useful data to the overcoming of central issues of principle or method' (Cattell 1946).

The concept of a trait is intimately related to that of correlation, and the statistical procedure underlying the work of the trait theorists is factor analysis. Charles Spearman first discussed factor theory around the turn of the century, though the matrix theory formulation of factor analysis did not really emerge until Thurstone's work in the 1930s. Factor analysis is, incidentally, one of the few scientific methodologies that psychology has been able to offer to other disciplines. The single most distinctive feature of factor analysis is its capacity to reduce a complex mass of data to a more simple and more orderly form. In the simplest design, one might measure a sample of people on a number of variables. The scores are then intercorrelated in every possible pairing to form a correlation matrix. Factor analysis is a technique which helps us to see whether there is some underlying pattern of relationships enabling us to reduce or to rearrange the data in such a way that a small set of factors can be extracted. Spearman's initial work on factorial methods was based upon the assumption that whenever two or more abilities are correlated, they can be regarded as depending upon a common factor. The factors that emerge may be taken as the source variables which account for the observed correlations in the data. The advantage of this procedure is obvious if there are a large number of initial variables. The intercorrelations among 100 variables would yield almost 5000 simple correlation coefficients, but could probably be reduced quite effectively to about 10 factors.

Factor analysis has an especially useful place in the early stages of research when basic concepts are still lacking. Until the important variables have been identified, the design of experiments remains largely a matter of trial and error, and there is little hope of working out any precise laws about the relationships between variables. Cattell (1952) has stressed this role of factor analysis in finding the independently-acting influences before moving on to experimentation, and factor theorists in general have emphasised the importance of factor analysis as a technique for the identification of the inherent organisation or *structure* in complex sets of data.

7.1 Guilford

Probably the first attempt to apply factor analytic methods to personality questionnaire data was that of Guilford, whose work influenced both Cattell and Eysenck. The study of Guilford and Guilford (1934) showed no single factor common to all test items, but a number of common factors emerged. These were tentatively identified as (a) social introversion-extraversion, (b) emotional sensitivity, (c) impulsiveness and (d) interest in self. This analysis was later repeated using more refined factor analytic techniques, and three main factors were found (Guilford and Guilford 1936). These were labelled S for social shyness, E for emotional immaturity or emotional dependency, and M for masculinity. Later research isolated further factors, and on the basis of a very large factor analysis Guilford and Zimmerman (1956) confirmed all the 13 factors hypothesised by Guilford.

Guilford's main factors:

G. General Activity. Fast-moving, energetic, drive for activity, feelings of adequacy and self-confidence, impulsiveness.

A. Ascendance. Standing up for one's rights, social leadership, liking to be conspicuous, taking the initiative.

M. Masculinity versus Femininity. Has masculine interests, not emotionally excitable or expressive, not easily aroused to fear or disgust, somewhat lacking in sympathy.

I. Confidence versus Inferiority Feelings. Feelings of acceptance, social poise, *versus* self-centred, discontent, fear of social contacts, ideas of reference, guilt and restlessness.

N. Calmness versus Nervousness. Nervous, easily tired, restless, tense, easily annoyed or depressed.

S. Sociability. Enjoys friends and social events, takes the role of leader, gregarious.

T. Reflectiveness. Enjoys serious thinking and introspection. Meditative and day-dreaming.

D. Depression. Emotional depression, physical tiredness, anxious, emotionally labile and lonely.

C¹ Emotionality. Emotions easily aroused and perseverating. Emotionally immature, wanting sympathy and fault-finding towards others.

R. Restraint. Not spontaneous or carefree, serious and avoids action and excitement.

O. Objectivity. Realistic, objective, not suspicious or hypersensitive.

Ag. Agreeableness. Friendly and compliant. Low scorers show resistance to control, contempt for others, suspiciousness, doubts about the honesty of others, hostility and aggression.

Co. Co-operativeness. Low scorers are fault-finding, suspicious, hostile, self-pitying and egocentric.

There is a considerable degree of overlap between these primary traits; they are not separate and independent. The correlation between N (Calmness) and D (Depression), for instance, is -0.44. Guilford rejected the use of an oblique rotational solution which makes it impossible to carry out a further factoring of the intercorrelations between the primary factors. The main factors include several which might be expected to relate to the neurotic disorders. The most relevant factors would perhaps be Depression (D) and Nervousness (N), though Emotionality (C^1) might also relate to some of the anxiety neuroses, and Restraint (R) could be expected to relate to obsessional and compulsive disorders. There is, however, no general, higher-order factor of neuroticism in Guilford's factor solution.

7.2 Cattell

Factor analytic studies of personality traits are largely based upon questionnaire data. Like Guilford, Raymond Cattell made extensive use of questionnaire data, but he also supplemented his investigations with data derived from objective tests (T-data), such as blood pressure and GSR measures, and from behaviour ratings taken from everyday life (life-record data or L-data). Although questionnaire data (Q-data) provide much of the basis for trait factor analytic studies, Cattell makes clear the limitations of such information. Personality questionnaires have a valid place in research, but the ease with which they can be abused has led to a seemingly endless stream of trivial articles: 'As a serious approach to discovering the structure of personality it [the excessive reliance upon personality questionnaires] represents the nadir of scientific inventiveness and subtlety' (Cattell 1946, p 341). Questionnaire data may be seen as existing in a world of its own, and there has been comparatively little research aimed at establishing the relationship of questionnaire data to overt behaviour.

Table 4. Cattell's first-order factors which discriminate between clinically judged neurotics and normals

Factor	Neurotic loading
Q4	High levels of tension and frustration
O	Prone to feelings of guilt, worry and remorse
F	Depressed and lethargic
I	Emotional sensitivity, tender-minded, unable to face emergencies
C	Low ego strength, emotional maladjustment and dissatisfaction
L	Suspicious, jealous, wary of others, rigid defences
E	Dependent and submissive
H	Easily threatened, timid, withdrawn

In the analysis of data derived from different sources, Cattell obtained much the same results with Q- and L-data, but found no simple one-to-one relationship between the factors derived from Q- and L-data and those from T-data. As a result, Cattell's system is extremely complex, since it contains primary factor solutions for all three types of data, as well as second-order factor solutions. The primary trait factors (derived from Q- and L-data) which relate to such aspects of neurosis as excessive worrying, irrational emotionality, feeling of inadequacy, hypochondria, low self-image, phobic, compulsive and somatic symptoms are shown in Table 4. Each of these factors discriminates significantly between clinically judged neurotics and normal subjects. As in Guilford's system, there is no single neuroticism factor, and Cattell has stressed the need for a multifactor theory to cover the various manifestations of neurosis (Cattell and Scheier 1961).

Second-order factors are broader dimensions which often correspond more closely to common clinical concepts and permit discussion in terms of fewer categories. Cattell recognised these higher-order factors as representing broader and more general features of personality structure, but because of this he saw them as failing to account for as much of the variance in specific behavioural events. The second-order factors that can be used to discriminate between neurotics and normal subjects are *F (Q) II, Anxiety,* (clinically judged neurotics are very much more anxious than normals) *and F (Q) IV, Resignation* (neurotics are more likely to score low on measures of dominance and assertiveness). The two remaining second-order factors approach, but just fail to achieve, statistically significant levels in discriminating between neurotic and normal groups. These are *F (Q) I,* Invia-Exvio (clinically judged neurotics tend to be more introverted than normal subjects) and *F (Q) III,* Pathemia (neurotics show more evidence of emotional immaturity and irrational hypersensitivity). As with the primary factors, Cattell finds no single factor at the second-order level which is adequate to distinguish between neurotic and normal groups; each of the factors is in some way essential to the definition of the neurotic condition.

In the analysis of behavioural test (T-) data a number of investigations showed a single anxiety-related factor at the first-order level. This contrasts with the several different primary factors of this sort that emerged from the analysis of Q- and L-data (Cattell 1957b). The single, general anxiety factor *(UI 24),* which emerged from the behavioural and physiological measures, corresponds closely to the clinician's unitary concept and has been identified as free-floating manifest anxiety. It includes such diverse manifestations of anxiety as irritability, emotionality, self-criticism, tremor and reduced salivary secretion. The concept of neurosis has traditionally been supposed to be closest to anxiety, and neurotics do score highest on UI 24. Using this factor as a marker, Scheier (1972) ranked some 20 clinical groups comprising over 2000 cases. The highest scores were recorded for anxiety states (90th percentile), reactive depression (85th percentile), obsessive-compulsive neuroses (75th percentile) and conversion reaction (70th percentile). The anxiety scores for psychosomatic disorders (in males) were much lower (50th percentile). Nonetheless, neurotics also score highly on five or six other factors in Cattell's system, and neurosis cannot be regarded as synonymous with UI 24: it is a composite of several factors, of which UI 24 is only one. Cattell (1957b) found a seperate factor of neuroticism which is quite distinct from the general anxiety factor and which also discriminates between neurotic and normal groups. This factor (UI 23) is characterised predominantly in terms of lack of ego strength. This neurotic debility is distinct from the actual neurotic behaviour which is determined partly by specific environmental stressors and by the pre-neurotic personality. Cattell refers to this factor as 'the essential ego weakness' which shows itself in a varity of defence mechanisms, emotional instability and feelings of inadequacy (Cattell op. cit.).

In the case of the anxiety factor, there remains the problem that analyses based upon L- and Q-data fail to show any general primary factor of the sort that emerged from analyses of T-data. However, the second-factor analyses established the higher-order anxiety factor, F (Q) II (Cattell 1957b; Cattell and Scheier 1961). This factor is characterised by weak ego-strength (H−), suspicion (L+), guilt-proneness (O+), low self-sentiment (Q3−) and tenseness (Q4+). This higher-order *Anxiety versus Dynamic Integration* factor may be identified with the general anxiety factor (UI 24) derived from T-data. When Q- and T-measures have been used together, the second-order Q- and the first-order T-pattern have emerged in the same factor. The most highly loaded primary factor in this second-order questionnaire factor is Q3 (−), which may also be regarded as the essential component of the higher-order factor. Q3 has been interpreted through its content and associations as an expression of the strength with which the individual strives to behave in accordance with a realistic and consciously approved self-image, and Cattell (1957b) regards this factor as an indication of how anxiety is the result of a failure of the dynamic integration of personality and behaviour.

It is interesting that Cattell sees the high loading of ergic tension (Q4) on the anxiety factor as supportive of Freud's (1936) suggestion that anxiety should be proportional to id pressure; 'Anxiety is ergic tension out of control' (Cattell 1957b). He also discusses the relationship between low ego strength (C−) and anxiety in terms of Freudian theory, though it is by no means clear what sort of relationship exists between the two. It is possible that the weak ego responds to threat by generating anxiety, or that high levels of anxiety, especially during early periods of development, lead to an impoverished self-image. However, the three factor psychosexual theory of personality proposed by Freud (oral, anal and phallic characters) bears little ressemblance to Cattell's system, and neither Cattell's primary-, nor his secondary-factor solutions can be said to provide direct support for Freudian theory (Cattell and Kline 1977).

7.3 Eysenck

In contrast to both Guilford and Cattell, Eysenck has always stressed the importance of a general factor of neuroticism. Eysenck (1967) suggests that the widespread use of the general concept of 'neurosis' reflects a universal recognition that there is something common to each of the specific neurotic disorders, and that it is this common 'something' that emerges from the factor analyses as neuroticism. Earlier concepts of this kind were described by McDougall in his 'self-regarding sentiment', and both Janet's 'misere psychologique' and Pavlov's notion of 'strength of nervous functioning' have some resemblance to Eysenck's neuroticism factor (Eysenck 1947a, b). Eysenck refers to the higher-order factors in his system as 'types', by which he means concentrations of correlated traits (Eysenck 1970b). As such, the difference between the concepts of type and trait lies not in the continuity or the discontinuity of the hypothesised variable, nor in its form of distribution, but in the greater inclusiveness of the type concept. Unfortunately, the notion of types continues to carry implications of discontinuity, and for the present discussion we will refer instead to higher-order trait factors. Eysenck has made extensive use of hierarchical models to illustrate the different levels of generality involved in his personality system, and a hierarchical model of the neuroticism factor is shown in Fig. 6.

Although Guilford and Cattell's trait factors clearly have some relationship to the neuroses, they were more interested in primary factors than general higher-order trait factors (Eysenck's type factors). As a result, their multifactorial questionnaires are difficult to relate directly to the clinical phenomena of neuroses. Eysenck, however, has attempted to do this and developed a series of questionnaires. The first such inventory, The Maudsley Medical Questionnaire, was succeeded by the Maudsley Personality Inventory (MPI), the Eysenck Personality Inventory (EPI) and, most recently, the Eysenck Personality Questionnaire (EPQ).

Eysenck's studies (1947a, 1970) have offered substantial support for the view that there are two separate and independent dimensions of neuroticism and psychoticism, both of which could be regarded as continuous with normality. For this reason, it was necessary to modify the earlier questionnaires to include a measure of psychoticism (P) as well as the measures of neuroticism (N) and extraversion (E) that were contained in the MPI and EPI. This was done in the EPQ (Eysenck and Eysenck 1975), which contains measures of N, P and E. Each of these scales provides a measure of an underlying personality trait which is assumed to be present to some degree in everyone (in normal groups the terms emotionality and tough-mindedness can be substituted for the psychiatric terms neuroticism and psychoticism).

Guilford, Cattell and Eysenck all rely heavily upon factor-analytic methods in their personality research, though factor analysis plays a lesser role in Eysenck's work. To him it remains an introductory tool which can be used in the primary, descriptive function of scientific enquiry, but which needs to be integrated with the main body of experimental and theoretical psychology. Eysenck has been emphatic about the importance of linking empirical research to a theoretical framework.

Despite the apparent differences in their work, there are a number of important areas of agreement in the factor solutions of these three workers, though these only appear in the higher-order factors. Guilford and Cattell have argued that a profile of many primary personality factors has more practical value than a small number of higher-order factors. On this point they disagree with Eysenck. Cattell, for instance, stated that first-order

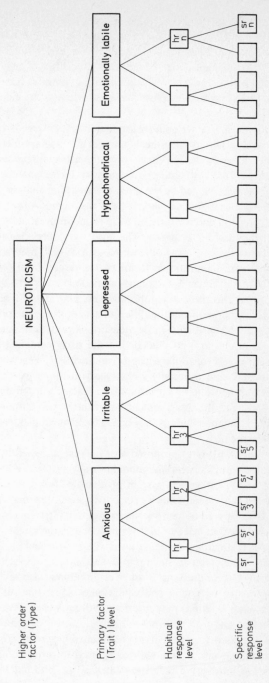

Fig. 6. The structure of Eysenck's concept of neuroticism

factors (and in particular the first-order factors derived from objective test data) provide at least as much information as any of the higher-order factors (Cattell and Scheier 1961). Eysenck, on the other hand, has argued that it is the higher order factors that have most psychological significance, and that little, if any, information is lost from the primary factors (Eysenck 1972). In addition, Eysenck has suggested that primary factors are not always replicable across the sexes, whereas the higher-order factors are replicable in this way.

The higher-order neuroticism factor that emerges from the questionnaires of all three authors is virtually identical, though the primary-factor solutions have comparatively little in common. The most comprehensive discussion of these issues (Eysenck and Eysenck 1969) is based upon a massive factor-analytic study of the questionnaire items and factors selected by the three authors. The analysis was conducted independently for the male and female samples. At the highest-order factor level, the two factors of extraversion and neuroticism were found in the male sample. In the female group, three separate factors emerged. The first two were clearly extraversion and neuroticism, whereas the third was difficult to identify and may have been largely an artifact. The higher-order neuroticism factor that emerged from combined analysis of the Guilford, Cattell and Eysenck factors contained all the items that had been identified with this factor in the three separate analyses, and at the higher-order factor level, the same factors emerged from the different sets of data. The primary factors, on the other hand, were not replicable from the questionnaire data of one investigator to another.

Adcock (1965) concluded that the disagreement between Cattell and Eysenck was based largely on differences of methodology regarding the number of factors to be extracted, and especially with regard to the question of rotation. Eysenck's centroid factor of neuroticism corresponds to Cattell's important second-order factor of anxiety. In this light, the disagreement between the two authors is more apparent than real, and Cattell's factor solutions may be regarded as supplementary rather than opposed to those of Eysenck.

Eysenck (1960c) proposed that his system, whereby the various neurotic groups are located within a two-dimensional framework (N × E) be used as a more reliable alternative to the categorical system of classification currently used in psychiatric diagnosis. Within this dimensional system, it is suggested that all neurotics score highly on the personality trait of neuroticism or emotionality. This N factor would appear to be essentially an emotional sensitivity which makes the person vulnerable to stress. The high N scorer is described as being an anxious, worrying person, prone to moods and depressions. He is likely to sleep poorly and suffer from various psychosomatic disorders. The dominant characteristic is an over-emotional disposition which responds strongly to a wide range of stimuli and which takes some time to return to normal. These strong emotional reactions may interfere with an appropriate adjustment to the person's environment and lead to irrational or rigid forms of behaviour. The second dimension (E) may be used to differentiate between different neurotic groups. Those whose central nervous system is innately predisposed towards excitation rather than inhibition will develop introverted patterns of behaviour, and patients suffering from anxiety states, reactive depression, phobias, obsessions or compulsive disorders tend to have high introversion scores: these are the dysthymic disorders. A combination of high N, high E, on the other hand, is likely to lead to 'psychopathic' and hysterical disorders. This involvement of extraversion with neuroticism was suggested earlier by Carl Jung, who proposed that in the case of a neurotic breakdown, extraverts were predisposed towards hysteria and psychasthenia. Eysenck is fond of tracing this notion even further back to Galen's doctrine of the four humours, particularly in the form given to it by Immanuel Kant (e. g. Eysenck 1957). Within this system, the dysthymic neurotic suffering from anxiety, depression, obsessions, or phobias would be expected to fall into the melancholic quadrant, with the hysterical disorders in the choleric quadrant.

It would be unwarranted, however, to assume that trait scores provide a direct measure of personality structure (Eysenck 1967). This is well illustrated by the results of Ingham's (1966) follow-up study. A group of 119 dysthymic and hysterical neurotic patients were retested 3 years after leaving hospital. The mean N scores of patients showing most improvement had declined, and the N scores for patients who showed the least improvement were almost unchanged. It was also found that the mean E scores of the most improved group had increased (again, those of the least-improved group were substantially the same). These findings suggest that trait-factor scores reflect changes in the symptomatic status of the patients and should be used only as indirect measures of the underlying personality structure.

Conditioning theory plays a central role in Eysenck's theory of neurosis, and it is predicted that introverts should condition more readily than extraverts. As a result, introverted subjects might be expected to acquire the conditioned fears and anxieties characteristic of the dysthymic states more easily than other people. The extraverted neurotic, on the other hand, is predicted to be vulnerable to hysterical disorders and to disorders of the second kind, such as nocturnal enuresis and the antisocial or psychopathic disorders (see Chap. 4). In these cases, it is suggested that there has been a failure of socially appropriate conditioning. The evidence on this point, however, is not entirely clear. Subjects who score high on N and low on E do appear to be more prone to dysthymic disorders, but hysterics, although high on N, are no more extraverted than normal groups (Eysenck 1967). It is possible that an excessive reliance on questionnaire measures may give a misleading impression, and Eysenck and Claridge (1962) conducted an investigation of normal subjects, dysthymic and hysterical neurotics, using four objective laboratory tests (sedation threshhold, two choice reaction task measures, and spiral after-effects) as well as questionnaire measures. A multiple discriminant function analysis was carried out, and two significant latent routes corresponding to N and E were extracted. The hysterics were the most extraverted group and the dysthymics the most introverted; on the neuroticism or emotionality variate, the normal subjects were the least neurotic.

The relationship of high N, low E to the dysthymic neuroses relates to the work on 'manifest anxiety', since the Manifest Anxiety Scale (Spence 1964; Taylor 1953) is loaded on both of Eysenck's dimensions of introversion and neuroticism (Eysenck 1965). Therefore, both Eysenck and Spence would agree (though for different reasons) that those individuals scoring high on this trait of manifest anxiety could be expected to form conditioned responses more readily than low scorers. Gray (1970b) has plotted the manifest anxiety scale against Eysenck's factors and suggests that the MAS covers the range from stable extraversion to introverted neuroticism (i. e. it indicates the most rapid increase in susceptibility to punishment).

Although Eysenck's theory works quite well for the dysthymic neuroses, the prediction that individuals who behave in a criminal or psychopathic manner should score highly on E and N must be regarded as unconfirmed. Although a number of studies (summarised in

Eysenck and Rachman 1965; Eysenck 1967) did find that criminals score high on both these dimensions, other studies have failed to find any evidence that such individuals are likely to be extraverted. Hoghughi and Forrest (1970) reviewed a number of studies of young offenders which consistently found them to be more introverted than the population norms or than selected control groups. Other studies of drug addicts found comparatively low E scores, even among addicts with high levels of antisocial and criminal behaviour in areas unrelated to drug abuse (Gossop 1978a, b; Gossop and Kristjansson 1977). With respect to antisocial forms of behaviour and criminality, therefore, Eysenck's predictions have not been unequivocally supported by the research findings.

7.4 Criticisms of Trait Theory

It is one of the most ancient psychological beliefs that there are pervasive consistencies in an individual's behaviour that show themselves across different situations. This assumption has been strongly challenged by several psychologists over the years. The earliest challenge came from the Hartshorne and May studies of moral behaviour in children (Hartshorne and May 1928; Hartshorne et al. 1929), which concluded that such traits as deception, helpfulness, co-operativeness, persistence and self-control were better seen as groups of specific habits rather than as general traits. In recent years, there has been a revival of criticism against the assumption of consistency in personality theory. Mischel (1968, 1977) has been one of the major figures in this debate and has argued that individuals show far less cross-situational consistency in their behaviour than has been assumed by trait theorists (and by personality theorists in general). Mischel suggested that the correlation coefficients of around +0.30 that have been commonly found for the consistency of behaviour across different situations reflect true behavioural variability rather imperfect measurement techniques. Correlations of this size account for less than 10% of the variance, and Mischel suggests that their value for making any predictive statements about behaviour is severely limited. This is a particular problem for the clinician who is primarily concerned with individual assessment and treatment issues. However, such correlations are fundamentally ambiguous. They can be used to support the trait theory position or to point to the specificity of behaviour in different situations.

Mischel's criticisms have been mistakenly seen as the expression of a hard-line environmentalist position which denies the existence of trait factors and attempts to replace them with situational and environmental factors as the basic units of study. This is not the case. Nor do trait theorists dismiss situational factors. Endler and Hunt (1969), for instance, differentiated between situationally-evoked anxiety and the trait of anxiousness. The S-R Inventories of traits were explicitly designed to separate situations from the modes of response which serve as indicators of reactions, states or traits. Trait anxiety may be regarded as the typical or chronic level of anxiety. Cattell described trait anxiety as a relatively permanent characteristic of individuals, and momentary state anxiety as a condition which varies from day to day or from moment to moment and which reflects the changes that occur in the person's environment (Cattell and Scheier 1961; Cattell and Kline 1977).

Objectively, state anxiety can be characterised by loadings on such physiological variables as high systolic blood pressure, raised body temperature, low basal skin resistance, increased heart rate, and in Q-data, state anxiety correlates with feelings of inability to cope. Cattell and Kline (1977) also offer an empirical distinction between trait and state anxiety in terms of the lower scores on protension (L), guilt (O) and responsiveness to threat (H) in state anxiety, though they point to some of the difficulties in maintaining this distinction between the two; (e. g. how long can a state last before it should be regarded as a trait?). Spielberger, who focused conceptual attention on this distinction between traits and states, reported correlations of $+0.44$ and $+0.67$ between his A-trait and A-state scales (Spielberger et al. 1968), and it has been suggested that both might fall largely within Cattell's UI 24 factor: that is, they could be regarded as functionally equivalent (Scheier 1972). There is a tendency in Cattell's work to incorporate environmentally-dependent states within the personality sphere, as when he argues for the existence of *state-liability traits* corresponding to each particular state (Cattell and Kline 1977). This tendency to overrate the importance of traits at the expense of environmental factors has been one of the prime complaints of the social-cognitive learning theorists.

Nevertheless, it would be equally mistaken to overrate situational factors or to set up pseudo-issues concerning the relative importance of persons versus situations. In one study of anxiety (Endler and Hunt 1966), it was found that neither individual differences nor situational factors alone contributed more than 4% to 6% of the total variance. The specific types of behavioural response, on the other hand, accounted for as much as 25% of the variance, and almost one-third of the variance came from simple interaction effects (subjects $\times$ situations, subjects $\times$ modes of response and situations $\times$ modes of response). The authors suggest that anxiousness is idyosyncratically organised, and that the validity coefficients for questionnaire measures of anxiety would probably be raised by specifying the sort of situations in which response measures of anxiety are to be reported.

Another modification of the trait theory approach is that of Bem, who suggests that the low correlations between trait measures and behaviour, as in the Hartshorne and May studies, show that people are not consistent in the same way as each other, but not that people are inconsistent with themselves. Trait research will only provide evidence of cross-situational consistency if the individuals in the research share the investigator's view of the equivalence of behaviours and situations. Those individuals who identify themselves as being consistent with regard to a particular trait (e. g. anxiousness, introversion, friendliness) will be more consistent in the way they behave in different situations than others who see themselves as highly variable (Bem and Allen 1974). This cognitive reinterpretation of trait theory has certain similarities to George Kelly's (1955) personal construct theory, in which the individual is allowed to generate his own trait-like constructs to characterise himself and his social world. The value of this self-attribution approach to the neuroses has been shown in the recent study of depression by Lewinsohn et al. (1979).

Few (if any) psychologists would deny that behaviour is dependent upon a complex interaction of factors. Trait theorists as well as social-cognitive theorists agree on this point. No trait theorist has asserted that such complex forms of behaviour as the neurotic disorders are a result of personality factors alone. Cattell and Kline (1977) specify an equation, which, whatever its other limitations, includes stimulus, response and situational factors, together with trait factors as multiple determinants of behaviour. They also take account of cognitive factors (viz. the individual's perceptions). To this extent, the disagreement between the social-cognitive and trait theorists is essentially one of the *relative utility* of trait and cognitive formulations in the clinical context (Certainly this seems to have been one of Mischel's primary concerns in *Personality and Assessment*).

The events that occur in the outside world and the phenomena that are studied by psychologists can be categorised and interpreted in many alternative ways. The number of alternatives is limited only by the investigator's inventiveness. The choice between the available alternatives is guided not by some absolute criterion of truth or reality but by assessing their usefulness, which in turn depends upon the investigator's purposes. This question of the utility of trait theory and social-cognitive approaches to clinical problems has been consistently stressed by Mischel (1968, 1973, 1979). Traits are useful as charac- terisations of what people are like 'in general', and as such they may show considerable reliability and stability over a period of time. At lower and more specific behavioural levels, however, categorisations tend to show the discriminativeness of behaviour in relation to different situations and give greater weight to the within-individual variance in behaviour than to measures of central tendency (Mischel 1979).

For the particular purposes of the clinician, it has been suggested that generalised traits may be too crude and gross as units for the analysis of complex behaviour, and that non- cognitive personality dispositions have far less effect upon behaviour than both trait and psycho-dynamic personality theorists have assumed (Mischel 1969). Trait theory formu- lations may even have helped to obscure the situational-specificity of behaviour in the attempt to demonstrate cross-situational generality. Ajzen and Fishbein (1977) have shown that the best predictors of a given behaviour are likely to be tailored to that specific behaviour. Equally, for clinical purposes (e. g. in setting up an individual treat- ment programme) an analysis of specific behaviours as they occur in a specific context is likely to be more useful than knowledge of the individual's position on one or more trait dimensions. Against this, it has been argued that trait theory is not intended to be used for the prediction of specific behaviours, but for wider scientific purposes of personality description.

A less tangible benefit of these social-cognitive criticisms is that they may help to correct the mechanistic view of human behaviour that is sometimes associated with other theories. Explanatory frameworks that are based upon stimulus-response theory, trait theory or psycho-analytic theory sometimes appear to imply that human action is the passive product of processes or forces over which the individual has no control. This can be seriously misleading. The child's ability to delay gratification, for instance, is clearly related to the cognitive strategies that he or she uses: the person's interpretation of his environment has a powerful effect upon the way that the environment will influence him (Mischel 1973). Even in areas such as drug addiction, where the individual appears to act under compulsion and might therefore be expected to have less control over his own behaviour, the person's attitudes, beliefs and expectations remain important factors (Eiser 1979; Gossop 1979).

8. The Physiology and Genetics of Neurosis

8.1 Physiology and Neurosis

Emotional states may be gauged in terms of the subjective experiences of the individual, his behavioural responses and his physiological reactions. Fear, for instance, has been described as an amalgam of apprehension, autonomic disturbances and avoidance behaviour (Rachman 1974); and these three components are now known to show some degree of independence (Rachman and Hodgson 1974). The physiological components of neurosis have always been important, both to our understanding of the neuroses and as a pointer to the physiological bases of personality.

The principal feature of the emotional states that distinguishes them from other mental phenomena is the extent to which autonomic arousal is an integral part of the emotions (Sartory and Lader 1980). Most psychophysiological responses associated with the emotions originate in the autonomic nervous system (ANS). This is divided into the sympathetic and para-sympathetic systems. The brain centre most importantly involved in the activation and regulation of these systems is the hypothalamus: the posterior hypothalamus primarily activates the sympathetic system, and the anterior hypothalamus, the para-sympathetic system. Strong sympathetic arousal is often indicated by increased heart rate and breathing, increased systolic blood pressure, dryness in the mouth and increased sweating.

In addition to producing a general sympathetic response, activation of the posterior hypothalamus leads to the release of hormones which stimulate the pituitary gland to secrete adrenocorticotrophic hormone (ACTH) into the blood stream: this hormone in turn causes the adrenal gland to secrete adrenocortical hormones (ACH). These latter hormones appear to help the organism in its response to stress, and the interaction of these two glands is generally referred to as the *pituitary-adrenal axis*.

When exposed to a wide range of stressful stimuli (whether emotional or physical) for a prolonged period of time, the pituitary-adrenal axis responds with certain distinctive changes. The sensitivity of the sympathetic-adrenomedullary system to certain psychological stimuli was investigated by W. B. Cannon during the early part of the century and this led to the 'emergency function' theory of adrenomedullary activity. More recently, Fahrenberg (1977) suggested that high levels of ACH excretion may indicate an alarm reaction as well as a constitutional hyper-reactivity of neuro-endocrine mechanisms; and low excretion levels may point to stability as well as exhaustion. The interpretation of such measures will depend upon knowledge of other factors.

Hans Selye's study of the body's responses to stress led to the formulation of the General Adaptation Syndrome (GAS) (Selye 1957). This emphasised the general, non-specific nature of the reactions. Selye suggested that many morphological, functional and

biochemical changes are common to the stress reaction, irrespective of the specific elicit-
ing stimulus. The three phases of the GAS were the alarm reaction, in which the body's
defences were mobilised, the stage of resistance, in which the body attempts to adapt to
the stress and finally, the stage of exhaustion. This stress syndrome was seen as
pathogenic, and Selye (1950) noted the striking similarity between the GAS and the
combat neuroses observed in soldiers during prolonged exposure to the stresses of warfare. Under extreme conditions of this sort, a whole range of psychosomatic disorders
may emerge, including disturbances of cardiac rhythm and blood pressure, excessive
sweating, bodily aches and pains, dizziness and fainting, paraesthesias, loss of libido or
impotence in the male, insomnia at night coupled with sleepiness during the day, morbid
fears, depression and compulsive thinking. Selye suggested that disorders of this sort are
fairly typical of the body's response to any prolonged systemic stress.

Despite the early excitement about the GAS, it has received much less attention in
recent years. It seems increasingly likely that the body's physiological reactions to stress
are not so general as Selye suggested, and the notion of stress is itself surrounded by a
number of conceptual problems. Lader (1975), for instance, suggested that 'the concept
of stress is so diffuse as to be not merely meaningless but even misleading.'

There have been other interesting studies of this problem of how the adrenomedullary
system responds to stressful stimuli. Weiss et al. (1976), for instance, proposed an alternative explanation for the learned helplessness findings. Under experimental conditions
in which they could not control shock, animals showed more severe gastric lesions,
greater loss of body weight, higher plasma steroid levels and more fearfulness than
controls (Weiss 1968). Overmier and Seligman (1967) stressed the escape-avoidance
learning deficit of animals exposed to inescapable shock, but argued that there was no
necessary connection between the stress-induced physiological changes and the
behavioural (avoidance) deficit. In contrast to Seligman's learned helplessness explanation of depression, Weiss proposed that the observed behavioural deficits were directly
related to physiological changes.

In the Overmier and Seligman (1967) study it was found that the escape-avoidance
deficit which was present at 24-hour retesting had disappeared after 48 hours. This rapid
dissipation of the deficit is not typical of learned responses, and Weiss suggested that the
results were caused by some physiological imbalance which corrects itself with time.
After a series of experimental investigations, Weiss et al. (1976) proposed that endogenous noradrenaline is differentially affected under conditions of escapable and inescapable shock, with excapable shock producing higher levels. More pertinent to Weiss's case
were the findings that experimental conditions which seemed to involve helplessness
without any reduction of noradrenergic activity in the brain led to no escape-avoidance
deficit, and that conditions which did not involve helplessness but which did reduce
noradrenaline levels led to a similar deficit to that observed by Overmier and Seligman.
Inescapable shock appears to be an especially potent condition, since even a single
exposure was found to cause marked depletion of noradrenaline concentrations in the
hypothalamic telencephalic regions of the brain. In a further investigation, Weiss and his
colleagues administered a monoamine oxidase inhibitor to the experimental animals with
the purpose of preventing the degradation of monoamines consequent upon inescapable
shock. Such animals showed no behavioural deficit after the experimental session,
whereas controls who had not received the MAO inhibitor showed the usual escape-
avoidance deficit.

The authors concluded that the depressive phenomena described by Overmier and Seligman (1967) and by Seligman and Maier (1967) were not a result of learned helplessness as such, but of a disturbance of central catecholamines. In particular, Weiss's explanation emphasised the role of noradrenaline depletion as the principal determinant, though other neurotransmittors may also be involved.

Psychophysiology is concerned with those physiological activities which underlie or relate to psychological functions, and a considerable amount of research has been concerned with the somatic concomitants of the neurotic disorders, and in particular of anxiety. In an investigation of the psychophysiological correlates of morbid anxiety, Lader and Wing (1966) found that the basal skin conductance level and the number of spontaneous fluctuations in skin conductance were both higher in patients than in normal subjects at rest: spontaneous fluctuations were also more frequent for the anxious patients throughout the experiment. Other studies found significantly greater forearm blood flow among anxious patients at rest than in normal subjects (Kelly 1966; Kelly and Walter 1968), and Howe (1958) found palmar skin resistance levels at rest were lower (increased sweating) among patients with chronic anxiety states. Other findings include elevation of basal heart rate and blood pressure among anxious subjects (Lader and Wing 1966; Goldstein 1964). These results fit in with Malmo's (1957) suggestion that anxious patients are over-aroused.

It has been widely assumed that neurotics (particularly anxiety neurotics) are more 'emotional' and therefore more autonomically labile than normal groups. However, the results of studies in which subjects have been presented with stimulation have yielded directly conflicting results. One group of investigators found that highly anxious subjects were more reactive than normal subjects. Goldstein (1964), for instance, found that systolic and diastolic blood pressure, respiration rate and heart rate were all higher in anxious patients than controls, both at rest and in response to stress. Similarly, Malmo and Shagass (1952) investigated the changes in blood pressure in a group of psychoneurotic patients under stress. Their results suggest that blood pressure is elevated in neurotics when they are under stress, and that this may indicate a greater and more prolonged change of blood pressure in response to stress among neurotics than in normal subjects.

Wing (1964), on the other hand, presented a difficult task to a group of patients suffering from anxiety states and measured skin conductance, pulse rate and EMG (muscle tension). The task produced short-lived physiological disturbances in both patients and controls. On all three measures the patients' mean levels were higher than those of the controls before, during and after the task, though the controls showed more responsiveness to stimulation than the patients, particularly in the case of the EMG. Lader and Wing (1966) found that the psychogalvanic reflex was smaller in patients than for controls in response to stimulation, and Kelly and Walter (1968) also found that anxious patients showed less physiological response to stressful stimulation than controls: normal subjects showed the greatest percentage increases in forearm blood flow, heart rate and self-rated anxiety when compared with a variety of neurotic and other psychiatric groups. These authors suggest that it is not the neurotic's ability to feel anxious which is abnormal, but their inability to relax in the absence of threatening stimuli. In any case, the assumption that anxiety neuroses reflect an underlying emotional hypersensitivity would appear to be an over-simplification. Lader and Wing (1966) have argued that autonomic reactivity is inversely related to the basal levels of activity in the sympathetic nervous system, and that powerful stimuli tend to reduce the differences between anxious patients and normals.

A recent overview of the psychophysiological literature (Sartory and Lader 1980) pointed to the following conclusions: anxiety states, and neuroses characterised by fearfulness and anxiety, seem to involve increased heart rate and increased forearm blood flow. Studies of muscle tension have led to inconsistent findings, possibly because of differences in the experimental methodologies, and different indices of electrodermal activity have also produced different results. Skin conductance level itself is a comparatively crude measure which only differentiates extreme groups, and skin resistance response is a complicated measure which probably represents an orienting reaction. Measures of spontaneous fluctuations in skin conductance may be a more valuable index of anxiety.

In other areas there is greater agreement in the experimental findings. It is clear that anxious patients take longer than normal both to adapt to changes in the experimental conditions and to habituate to stimuli. This has been found in psychophysiological studies of blood pressure (Malmo and Shagass 1952), GSR (Lader and Wing 1966) and EMG (Davis et al. 1954).

One reason for some of the conflicting results may lie in the use of inadequately defined patient groups such as 'neurotics'. This category covers such a wide range of disorders that a more precise specification of the patient characteristics is necessary before the experimental results can be properly interpreted. Lader (1967, 1969) has cautioned against the assumption that neurosis has any functional unity, and the investigation of psychophysiological parameters has been quite valuable in this context.

In a study of 90 patients with various psychoneurotic disorders, Lader (1967) measured changes in skin conductance levels during sound stimulation, rate of habituation and spontaneous fluctuations. Patients with specific phobias were differentiated from those with other affective disorders (including patients with social phobias and agoraphobia). The specific phobics habituated rapidly and had fewer spontaneous fluctuations (lower arousal), and in this respect they were most like normal subjects. Among the other patient groups, levels of arousal were higher than normal, as would be expected for anxious subjects, though it is interesting that increased arousal was also found in the agoraphobic and socially phobic patients who were not actually in anxiety-provoking situations. In an investigation of the clinical implications of this finding, Lader et al. (1967) found that specific phobics differed from social phobics and agoraphobics on clinical grounds, with earlier age of onset of symptoms and lower debility. The specific phobics showed the best response to desensitisation both in terms of reduction of clinical symptoms and in improvement in social functioning, and the authors conclude that autonomic measures can be a valuable means of predicting treatment outcome among phobic patients. Kelly and Walter (1968) also found that chronically anxious patients could be distinguished from controls by measures of basal forearm blood flow. On this measure the mean score of the anxious patients was more than twice as high as that of normal subjects, and higher than all other diagnostic groups in the study (agitated and non-agitated depressions, schizophrenia, obsessional neurosis, phobic states, hysteria, personality disorder and depersonalisation disorders). Both Kelly and Walter (1968) and Lader (1967) suggested that phobic patients have the closest resemblance to normal controls, although different physiological measures were used in the two studies. In the

Kelly and Walter results, patients with phobic and chronic anxiety states differed on almost every measure used.

Another study of 240 patients with symptoms of neurotic anxiety or depression was conducted by Frith et al. (1978). This showed a close relationship between symptoms of anxiety and depression (both self- and observer-rated). On physiological measures, however, the two groups could be differentiated – the anxiety neurotics taking longer than the depressed neurotics to habituate to a novel stimulus. When variously treated with amitriptyline (a tricyclic antidepressant), diazepam (an anxiolytic), both drugs together, or a placebo, Frith and his colleagues found that amitriptyline gave greater benefit to the depressed patients than the other treatments. Unexpectedly, the antidepressant also gave greatest benefit to the anxious patients, though diazepam did produce some improvement among the anxiety cases in terms of their physiological response: their electrodermal habituation times increased. This suggests that diazepam may alter the peripheral signs of anxiety without having any necessary effect upon the more complex subjective and behavioural manifestations.

On the whole, the autonomic accompaniments of depression have been less well researched than those associated with anxiety. This is partly because depression cannot be experimentally induced in the same way as anxiety. A further problem is that depression seldom occurs without at least some anxiety, and this may itself produce some of the observed physiological changes. Shagass and Jones (1958) found that the sedation threshold was low in psychotic depression and high in neurotic depression. This finding supports the distinction between the two types of depressive disorder discussed earlier in the book. However, because barbiturate plasma levels after a given dose tend to be inversely related to muscle blood flow (which has already be shown to be associated with anxiety level), sedation threshold may be as much a measure of the state of the peripheral vascular system as of any central process (Lader and Noble 1975). Similar difficulties arise in the case of EMG and GSR recordings, both of which are known to be affected by anxiety.

8.2 Eysenck

Eysenck's theory of the neuroses requires two descriptive dimensions and probably two causal processes, both of which are closely linked to physiological and genetic factors. The dimension of neuroticism is conceived in terms of individual differences in the reactivity and lability of the autonomic nervous system, and the autonomic lability itself is seen as an inherited characteristic of the organism. Eysenck and Rachman (1965) suggest that some people are 'innately predisposed to respond more strongly, more lastingly, and more quickly with their autonomic nervous system' when presented with stressful stimuli.

This notion that neurotic patients (particularly those with anxiety neuroses) might suffer from some sort of autonomic lability or over-reactivity is not new. Many psychiatrists and psychologists with a physiological training have subscribed to this sort of view, and Cattell like Eysenck favours two distinct concepts of physiological arousal. The first is a general autonomic-endocrine activation which corresponds most closely to the anxiety trait factor UI 24 and to the anxiety state factor (SUI 9). This state anxiety factor is associated with raised heart and respiration rates, high systolic blood pressure, low resting skin resistance, low serum cholinesterase and high plasma 17-ketosteroids (Fahren-

berg 1977). Cattell also includes cortical arousal in his system. This corresponds mainly
to his UI 22 factor and closely resembles the concept of cortical arousal, which plays such
a central role in Eysenck's theory.

Eysenck's trait factor dimension, introversion-extraversion, is linked to the processes
of inhibition and excitation. Indeed, it is this dimension of introversion-extraversion and
the closely related concepts of inhibition and excitation that have received most attention
in Eysenck's work. (Inhibition and excitation are used here to refer to properties of the
central nervous system, and not to aspects of behaviour.) Extraverts are said to be
characterised by a predominance of inhibitory activity, and introverts by a predominance
of excitatory forces (Eysenck 1957). Eysenck formulates these effects in terms of reactive
inhibition – a concept which can be traced back through the work of Clark Hull to that of
Pavlov. In those people with an autonomic predisposition towards neurosis, it is this
balance of inhibitory and excitatory forces that determines the development of specific
neurotic symptoms. Like the autonomic lability which is the physiological substrate of N,
this balance of forces is also regarded as constitutionally inherited.

Individual differences in neuroticism are related to differential thresholds of arousal in
the visceral brain, and behavioural differences with respect to extraversion are related to
differential thresholds in various parts of the ascending reticular activating system
(ARAS). It is suggested that cortical arousal can be produced in two ways. It may be a
result of sensory stimulation or of higher mental processes, in which case there need be
no arousal of the viceral brain, or it may be produced by emotion. In this latter case, there
is both cortical and autonomic arousal. Autonomic activation and cortical arousal are,
therefore, partially independent, and Eysenck cautions against any assumption that such
measures of cortical arousal as EEG, GSR or EMG can be used as direct indices of
emotional involvement.

Eysenck provides support for his theory with evidence derived from a wide range of
experimental techniques, including sedation threshold, spiral after-effect and vigilance.
Extensive reviews of these findings are offered both by Eysenck (1967) and by Claridge
(1967). With respect to sedation threshold, for instance, Eysenck's theory predicts that
extraverts (and extraverted neurotics such as hysterics, psychopaths and personality disorders) would show *low* thresholds, and that introverts (and dysthymic neurotics) would
show *high* thresholds. This result was obtained by Shagass and Jones (1958) in a
neurophysiological investigation of different diagnostic groups. Patients with hysteria had
the lowest sedation threshold, followed by patients diagnosed as suffering from mixed
neurosis and anxiety hysteria (phobic disorders). The highest threshold was obtained for
patients with anxiety states, followed by neurotic depressives.

Similar supportive evidence has been obtained using the spiral after-effect. Duration of
the after-effect should be less in extraverts than in introverts because of the higher levels
of reactive inhibition in the former group, and although there have been a few failures to
confirm this effect, most studies did find the predicted differences between introverted
and extraverted subjects. Claridge (1967), however, has argued that Eysenck's excitation-inhibition hypothesis, insofar as it is linked to the single dimension of introversion-
extraversion (or to a single underlying causal process), is inadequate. Instead, Claridge
suggests that two dimensions are necessary to account for the results of experimental and
physiological studies with neurotic groups.

8.3 Claridge

Claridge's theory may be regarded as a reinterpretation of Eysenck's theory in arousal terms. Whereas Eysenck placed excitation and inhibition on a single dimension and described them as reciprocally related, Claridge suggests that two dimensions are required and that these are congruent in activity. Claridge (1960) suggests that Eysenck's introversion-extraversion and neuroticism dimensions are not functionally independent, and that *both* may be regarded as dimensions of arousal. On a number of objective tests, the performance of hysterics and dysthymics failed to match their scores on one of Eysenck's personality questionnaires (the MPI) (Claridge 1967). In a principal components analysis of the objective test data (e. g. sedation threshold and spiral after-effect) and of the questionnaire measures of extraversion and neuroticism, two correlated factors emerged; both were related to arousal. On the basis of these results, Claridge proposed a theory based upon two functionally related arousal mechanisms. The first is identified as a *tonic arousal system*. This maintains the individual's gross level of arousal. The second is described as the *arousal modulating system,* and its functions are to regulate the level of activity in the tonic arousal system and to integrate stimulus input into both systems. The two systems may be seen as related in such a way as to provide a negative feedback loop regulating the level of arousal.

Claridge, like Eysenck, is mainly concerned to explain the differences between hysteria and the dysthymic neuroses. But unlike Eysenck, Claridge proposed that where there are high levels of activity in the arousal modulating system, this leads simultaneously to high levels of inhibition in the arousal modulating system to match the high levels of activity in the tonic arousal system. In the dysthymic neuroses, high tonic arousal is matched by high levels of inhibition in the arousal modulating system. In the hysterical and psychopathic neuroses, the reverse is true. Tonic arousal and (inhibitory) arousal modulation are both at a low level.

One advantage of this theory is that it can account for the failure to find high E scores in hysterical and psychopathic groups (McGuire et al. 1963; Gossop and Kristjansson 1977; Hoghughi and Forrest 1970). On the other hand, Claridge's two dimensions and the hypothesised tonic arousal and arousal modulating systems are comparatively difficult to reconcile with physiological findings (as Claridge acknowledges). They operate at a conceptual and theoretical level rather than at the level of neuro-anatomy or physiology.

8.4 Gray

Gray (1972) has also proposed a psychophysiological theory of personality, which may be seen as an extension and modification of Eysenck's (1957, 1967) theory of introversion-extraversion. Instead of the ascending reticular activating system, Gray suggests that a more extensive system acts as the physiological substrate of introversion. This consists of the ARAS together with the medial septal area, the hippocampus and the orbital frontal cortex and their interconnections.

The barbiturate drugs and alcohol both antagonise the activity of the physiological system which Gray labels the punishment mechanism, without affecting the reward mechanism. Gray argues that the ARAS is unlikely to be the chief site of action for this sensitivity to specific types of reinforcement (i. e. reward or punishment), and the hippocampus and medial septal area are suggested as an alternative site of action. The behavioural effects of the barbiturates and alcohol seem to be due to an action on the septal mechanism for production of the hippocampal theta rhythm (Gray 1970a). More precisely, amobarbital appears to affect behaviour by antagonising the normal theta rhythm response to punishment and frustrative non-reward (Gray 1972). Whereas Eysenck (1957) links introversion to increased cortical arousal in the ARAS, Gray regards the level of introversion as determined by the amount of activity in the septo-hippocampal system. This operates as a negative feedback loop consisting of the orbital frontal cortex, the medial septal area and hippocampus as well as the ARAS.

Eysenck's theory places considerable weight upon the notion of conditionability as a general personality feature. This is attributed to the relatively high level of arousal in introverts who are regarded as over-socialized: (by socialization Eysenck primarily means the acquisition of conditioned fear responses; e. g. Eysenck 1960b). In addition, Eysenck uses the notion of general conditionability to account for the important behavioural and psychiatric differences between the dysthymic, and the hysterical and psychopathic disorders. However, it seems that introverts condition better than extraverts *only under certain conditions*. In general, introverts seem to condition better under conditions of under-arousal, whereas under conditions of over-arousal, extraverts perform comparatively well (Eysenck 1967).

There is a considerable body of evidence showing systematic differences in arousal between introverts and extraverts. However, after Seligman's (1970) discussion of the inadequacy of the general process view of learning, there is increasing doubt that con-ditionability can be regarded as a unitary concept. Since much of Eysenck's evidence rests upon the results of eye-blink conditioning studies, his theory would be considerably weakened by studies demonstrating the specificity of conditioned connections.

Gray (1970b) rejected Eysenck's conditionability interpretation of introversion and replaced the notion of conditionability (thought to be greater in introverts than extraverts) with that of susceptibility to punishment and frustrative non-reward. This is also supposed to be greater among introverted subjects. Because the introvert is more highly aroused, Gray (1972, 1976) regards him as more susceptible to punishment. Conversely, the extravert is described as being 'bad at fear' (Gray 1971). Gray has used this to explain, for instance, the psychopathic features of criminality and antisocial behaviour in the absence of anxiety or guilt, and the recidivism that accompanies psychopathic behaviour (Gray 1970b). Psychopathic behaviour is seen as the tendency of the extraverted neurotic to seek reward without fear of punishment, and the dysthymic symptoms of the introverted neurotic can usually be seen as a clear expression of fear. Even in the case of the obsessional who performs his rituals in a state of apparent calm, any interference with the obsessions is likely to cause overt and sometimes intense fear. On this point, Gray's theory runs into the same difficulties as that of Eysenck (see previous chapter): individuals who behave in a criminal or psychopathic manner do not consistently show high levels of extraversion.

8.5 Genetics and Neurosis

Virtually all psychologists recognise that individual differences are a salient feature of any behavioural analysis. On the question of whether or not there may be a genetic component underlying the observed individual differences, however, there is considerable (and often acrimonious) debate, though there has always been an interest in genetic determinants of the neurotic disorders. Maudsley (1899) commented: 'There is a destiny made for each man by his inheritance; he is the necessary organic consequent of certain organic antecedents', and Freud, in his *General Theory of the Neuroses* (1917), stressed the inherited component of libidinal development and referred to the hereditary sexual constitution. More recently, Eysenck & Cattell have been concerned with the genetic determinants of personality, and most psychologists with a biological training would be prepared to accept that a predisposition towards nervousness could be inherited.

The genotype (or the biological inheritance transmitted by genes) cannot be measured directly, and the phenotype (or observable characteristics of an individual) is not itself inherited. However, by selecting animals according to phenotype and mating like with like, it is possible to produce phenotypic differences. Broadhurst's selective breeding for extremes of emotionality in the rat led to the establishment of the Maudsley reactive and non-reactive strains (Broadhurst 1978). This emotionality factor may be comparable to the autonomic lability which has been suggested as an underlying determinant of human neuroticism (Eysenck 1967).

8.6 Studies of Twins

One of the most useful vehicles for the investigation of genetic effects is the study of twins. Its basic rationale was first propounded by Galton in 1875, and twin studies have been regarded as a sort of natural experiment allowing the differentiation of genetic and environmental influences. Identical (monozygotic) twins are born with identical genotypes, whereas in genetic terms, fraternal (dizygotic) twins are no more alike than ordinary siblings. Estimates of genetic effects are sometimes based upon the difference in correlation between identical and same-sex fraternal twins, though this method is not without its limitations, because of the possibility that environmental effects for identical twins may differ in subtle ways from those for other twins. Nonetheless, in studies of a particular trait or illness, results pointing to higher concordance rates in identical than in fraternal twins are suggestive of some underlying genetic factor. Another type of investigation has looked at the similarities between identical twins who have been reared apart.

Rutter et al. (1963) carried out a longitudinal study of the development from birth of 56 siblings and twins, in which several behaviour patterns (the authors refer to these as 'primary reaction patterns') were investigated. Evidence of genetic influence was obtained for most of these primary reaction patterns, though it is interesting that those categories in which the evidence for a genetic basis was strongest were also those showing the *greatest instability* over time. Among these, was the approach-withdrawal pattern, which may well be related to fearfulness, and which has been found to be a precursor of later childhood behaviour disorders (Thomas et al. 1968). Conversely, Rutter found that those patterns showing the greatest stability gave the least indication of genetic determination.

On autonomic measures, identical twins have been found to be more alike on measures of heart rate than fraternal twins (Vandenberg et al. 1965) and there is also a high degree of similarity between identical twins in terms of palmar skin resistance (Block 1967). Lader and Wing (1966) compared 11 pairs of monozygotic and 11 pairs of dizygotic twins on a number of physiological measures which differentiated between anxiety states and normals. On measures of the habituation of electrodermal response, a correlation of +0.75 was obtained for MZ, and +0.13 for DZ twins; the spontaneous GSR fluctuations towards the end of the experimental session correlated +0.68 for MZ twins and −0.02 for DZ twins; and pulse rate correlated +0.78 for MZ and −0.38 for DZ twins. The negative correlations obtained for the DZ group are puzzling. If a genetic factor is operative, correlations for the DZ group should be lower than for MZ subjects but they should still be positive. It is possible that this result is a reflection of error variance caused by the small groups used in the study.

This does not, however, alter the other findings, and the authors conclude that habituation of GSRs, the number of spontaneous fluctuations and pulse rate are subject to genetic influences. Another study of 84 male twins (Rust 1974) also reported a substantial genetic effect (of more than 60%) underlying electrodermal and heart rate basal measures, electrodermal response and spontaneous activity. This investigation failed to find any genetic component for habituation of electrodermal response, as in the Lader and Wing study.

Other studies of twins have used personality questionnaire data. On Cattell's High School Personality Questionnaire the results from over 100 MZ and 100 DZ pairs of twins suggest that there is greater resemblance between identical than fraternal twins on the General Neuroticism versus Ego-Strength Factor. Cattell and Scheier (1961) found that their main first-order anxiety factors were determined primarily by environmental rather than genetic factors, and in a study using the MMPI and HSPQ, Gottesman (1963) found comparatively low heritability indices for hypochondriasis and hysteria. This study did, however, report a substantial inherited component for social introversion (0.71), psychopathic deviation (0.50) and depression (0.45). The Introversion-Extraversion factor has consistently been found to have a considerable genetic component (Slater and Shields 1969). The results for neuroticism have been less consistent, though Shields (1962) found correlations of +0.38 on neuroticism for MZ twins reared together and +0.53 for twins reared apart. The correlation between N scores for DZ twins reared together was much lower (+0.11). An interesting feature of these results is that MZ twins reared apart appeared to be more similar on measure of neuroticism and extraversion than MZ twins reared together. It is not at all clear why this result was obtained, though it has also been reported in other investigations (e. g. Wilde 1964).

Clinical studies are undoubtedly hampered by the low reliability and validity of psychiatric diagnoses, but several interesting studies have been conducted in this area. If genetic factors contribute towards the determination of certain neurotic disorders, one might expect the relatives of neurotics to be more likely to show similar disorders. Brown (1942) looked at the incidence of neurotic disorders among the parents and siblings of anxiety neurotics, hysterics and obsessional neurotics. The incidence of neurosis among close relatives was found to be much higher than would be expected by chance, and there was marked variation in the tendency of first-degree relatives to share a similar diagnosis to the proband. For anxiety states 15.1% of the relatives were given the same diagnosis; for hysteria the rate was 11.2%, and 6.9% for obsessional neurosis. Unfortunately, there are massive problems involved in interpreting the results in studies of this sort. No correlation can be made for closeness of kinship and the expected rates for a given disorder, nor is there any control for environmental determinants. In addition, it is difficult to know whether or not experimenter bias may have distorted the results.

Slater and Shields (1969) reported a study of 146 cases who had been diagnosed as suffering from a neurotic or personality disorder and who had a twin partner. Of those individuals diagnosed as suffering from an anxiety state, 41% of the MZ twin partners were assigned the same diagnosis, against only 4% of the DZ twin partners. For the other neuroses (mostly reactive depressions), none of the twin partners received the same diagnosis. These results point towards some degree of genetic specificity for the anxiety states, but give no suggestion of genetic determination for the other neuroses. Neurotic depression, for instance, appears to have no specific genetic component, though there is some evidence that genetic factors do operate in endogenous or psychotic forms of depression.

In a review of ten studies of twins involving 1264 pairs of twins, Pollin (1976) noted that the concordance rates for neurosis between MZ twins were reliably found to be about twice as great as those for DZ twins. This increased tendency for both MZ twins to show signs of a neurotic disorder, although marked, was much less than the concordance rates found for schizophrenia. In this latter case, where one twin had a schizophrenic disorder, the MZ partner was $3^1/_2$–6 times more likely to have the same disorder than the DZ partner. These results suggest that some genetic component operates in the neuroses, but that there is a stronger genetic factor in the aetiology of schizophrenia.

The gist of these findings is that genetic factors appear to be involved in the determination of those neuroses which are primarily characterised by anxiety, but not in other neurotic disorders. It should not need to be restated that this does not imply that genetic factors may therefore be invoked as 'causes' of anxiety neuroses, or that environmental factors are of lesser significance.

It would be entirely futile to return to this sort of genetics *versus* environmental dichotomy, and several investigators have begun to express doubts about the utility of this general approach to the problem. Caspari (1967), for instance, suggests that questions of whether or not a given behaviour has a genetic component, or even how much of the variance can be attributed to genetic and environmental factors, may be misleading. A more appropriate formulation (especially for the clinical researcher) might ask how genetic individuality will express itself under varying environmental conditions. The majority of genetic studies have been concerned with estimates of *how much* a particular trait is inherited rather than with questions of *what* is inherited. Little is known about this, except that various polygenic systems seem to be involved, and it remains to be discovered how the genes exert their effect.

9. Overview

The concept of neurosis incorporates a group of disorders which are in many respects poorly defined and delineated. Nonetheless they are of great theoretical as well as clinical significance. If one accepts the estimate that as many as 13% or 14% of the general population may suffer from some form of neurotic disorder (Hagnell 1968; Shepherd 1973), it is clear that many millions of people are incapacitated to a considerable extent by the neuroses. Cattell and Scheier (1961) make an even higher estimate – that 25%–57% of the normal population will at some time be affected by a neurotic condition.

The American Psychiatric Association, in its recent attempt to rationalise the idea of neurosis, has abolished the term. There is no longer anyone in America who can be said to suffer from neurosis. However, the disorders that were previously subsumed within the general category of neurosis now re-appear in their separate and newly constituted roles in such subcategories as Anxiety Disorders (including phobias and obsessions), Somatoform Disorders (including conversion symptoms), Dissassociative Disorders (including amnesia and depersonalisation) and Post-Traumatic Reactive Disorders. When faced by the ambiguities and contradictions inherent in the current use of the term, it is understandable that the APA should have been tempted to abandon the general concept of neurosis. Concepts in science are not, however, replaced by executive decision (even when they are obviously unsatisfactory), but because they have been superseded by other more useful concepts.

It has been apparent for some time that the unitary concept of neurosis has quite obvious weaknesses. It lumps together disorders which are quite different in subjective experience, in their physiological concomitants and in their behavioural expression. One of the least useful features of the traditional concept of neurosis was the way in which it confused the descriptive and theoretical levels of discourse. Neurosis exists as a higher order concept which covers a variety of separate disorders with diverse symptomatic expressions, and it contains the implicit assumption that each of the disorders are connected in some way. This assumption operates in an insidious manner because it fails to specify the nature of the connection between the disorders.

It is important not to confuse the descriptive stage of research, in which we attempt to establish useful concepts, with the explanatory stage, in which we attempt to build theories to explain the phenomena covered by these concepts and bring together apparently diverse phenomena. It is essential to systems of classification that they should group phenomena according to their common features (Hempel 1961). But the fact that the neuroses share certain symptomatic similarities does not mean that they are necessarily the result of the same determinants. Equally, the symptomatic differences need not imply that different determinants were involved. The symptomatic expression of particular disorders exists at a descriptive level. The supposed connections between those disorders which are the essence of the higher-order concept of neurosis exist at a theoretical level. By making a more explicit separation of the neurotic disorders, DSM III may facilitate the observation and description of the separate disorders. But this will only be true if the classification system is treated as a descriptive system dealing with the symptomatic expression of the various neurotic conditions. This is unlikely to have been the intention of the APA, since the medical tradition requires diagnoses to go beyond description to make further statements about the causes of specific disorders as well as about their prognosis (Warner 1952; Kendell 1975).

It is improbable that each specific neurotic disorder will be found to have its own distinct determinants which set it apart from the other disorders. Most theories agree that anxiety is the central facet of neurosis. Freud's view after 1936 was that all of the psychoneuroses represented an attempt to avoid the conscious experience of anxiety. Neurotic anxiety was itself a response to some intrapsychic conflict: repression and the other mechanisms of this sort were motivated by the attempt to escape the conscious experience of this painful affect.

Although Eysenck's trait theory differs in most respects from Freud's system, this also regards the neuroses as sharing some common factor. Again this is closely linked to anxiety, but in this case through the proposed higher-order factor of neuroticism. All neurotics are said to score highly on this autonomic lability factor. Neuroticism is essentially a form of emotional sensitivity which makes the person unusually vulnerable to stress. Cattell's trait theory takes a different position. Again, anxiety is seen as the central feature of neurosis, but anxiety and neuroticism are clearly separated. Indeed, in Cattell's system, a range of factors are proposed, each of which is necessary to the understanding of neurosis. This multifactor theory stands in contrast to Eysenck's system, since neither at the first-order nor at the second-order level do neurotic patients differ significantly from normal subjects on only one central factor of neuroticism.

Anxiety, which is generally regarded as a central component of neurosis, may be usefully divided into its physiological, behavioural and cognitive components. Until recently, the emphasis upon behavioural and physiological features obscured the importance of the individual's cognitions. One of the most promising recent developments in abnormal psychology has been the interest in cognitive processes. A common weakness of several theories of neurosis has been their neglect or exclusion of the individual's attitudes, beliefs and intentions. It is now becoming increasingly apparent that the way in which the individual perceives himself, the objects and events in his environment and the meaning that he attaches to them are extremely important to our understanding of human behaviour. The classic series of experiments by Schachter and Singer (1962) showed how emotional states depend upon their meaning for the individual, and other investigators have shown how attribution processes can affect the neuroses. Storms and Nisbett (1970) used an attributional model to explain the results of their study on insomnia, and Valins and Nisbett (1971) extended this analysis to such other neurotic disorders as the phobias, depression and homosexual panic.

The challenge facing any complete account of neurosis, however, is that of the neurotic paradox. The neurotic seems to behave in a manner which leads to predominantly unfavourable consequences, and which even the neurotic individual himself may see as irrational and undesirable. Yet he seems unable to maintain any change from his neurotic patterns of behaviour. A cognitive account of neurosis faces special difficulties in attempting to explain this paradox in cognitive terms. Learning theorists such as Mowrer (1950) have explained it by reference to the way in which the neurotic avoids exposure to the fear-producing situation. This protects the conditioned fear response from extinction. To this account, Eysenck (1976) added the idea that anxiety has drive properties and therefore leads to an incubation effect in which the unreinforced conditioned response retains its strength, or even becomes more powerful.

Freud was also well aware of this paradox. From the beginning of his psychological studies he had been fascinated by the behaviour of the neurotic individual. This seemed to be inexplicable in terms of common sense, in terms of the patient's conscious wishes and in terms of the current state of medical and scientific knowledge. The psycho-analytic solution is unique in its proposal of three major provinces of the mind in which various dynamic forces operate. The presence of intrapsychic conflict, which is itself determined in a highly complex way by the structure of personality, establishes neurotic anxiety, and in the conflict of drives, the neurotic symptoms appear as a compromise solution. All neurotic reactions function primarily as a defence against the threat posed by this irrational anxiety. Freud's attempt to explain the neurotic paradox consisted of his attempt to show that the psycho-neuroses operated according to the laws of unconscious mental forces.

The neurotic paradox has been most thoroughly investigated with respect to the anxiety disorders, but depression is also surrounded by paradox. There is usually a large discrepancy between the individual's perceptions of himself and the objective facts, and, as with the anxiety disorders, depressive behaviour also seems to contradict the principle that the person might be expected to act in such a way as to increase his sources of satisfaction and to minimise his pain.

The complex mixture of symptoms found among neurotic depressives also argues against an atomistic approach which too readily rejects the higher-order concept of neurosis in favour of discrete categories. It is quite clear, for instance, that neurotic depression regularly occurs together with anxiety and with other neurotic traits and symptoms. Grinker et al. (1961) found that free-floating anxiety was an important part of the clinical concept of depression, and the diagnosis of neurotic depression may be dependent upon the patient's also showing signs of anxiety. In those cases in which the patient is only slightly depressed, the presence of anxiety greatly increases the probability that they will receive a diagnosis of depression.

Several authors have related the neuroses to the individual's social circumstances, including his socio-economic status. Brown and Harris (1978), for instance, found that depression was more common among working-class women and offered an explanation in terms of how certain social factors act as provoking agents in depression. Other factors have a protective function, and yet others make the person more vulnerable to particular stressful events. There has also been considerable interest, particularly among sociologists, in the way in which neurosis may be seen as an ascribed social role. Despite its weaknesses, this view has been a useful antidote to the intra-individual approaches of most psychological accounts, and it has drawn attention to the way in which the social meaning of neurosis plays a part in the determination of the neuroses. Parson's concept of the sick-role is one of the best-known examples of this sort, and even such an individual-oriented system as psycho-analysis has acknowledged that the sick-role (though it is not referred to in such terms) can play a part in maintaining neurotic behaviour. Freud (1933, vol XXII, p 142) for instance has commented that 'The ego will seek to turn even illness to its advantage'. In Freudian theory, however, this is clearly described as a secondary gain which may add to the primary and unconscious gains provided by the neurotic symptoms. In itself it is not thought to be sufficient to account for the development of the symptoms, and the relationship of the individual's self-perceptions to his social environment are not dealt with at any length.

Of the neurotic disorders in which there is often a strong element of secondary gain, and to which the sick-role may well be applicable, hysteria stands out. This is one of the most curious of the neuroses, and it occupies a unique place in the history of psychological medicine. It was one of the first of the neurotic disorders to be described, and the work of Briquet, Charcot, Janet and Freud in this area has undoubtedly had a profound impact upon current thinking in abnormal psychology. Nonetheless, like the concept of neurosis itself, hysteria remains a vague and indefinite sort of term.

Partly because of this, partly because of its pejorative implications, and partly because the incidence of hysteria in the general population seems to have declined over the past century, hysteria is not often made as a specific formal diagnosis in current psychiatric practice. Slater (1965) has argued that the concept of hysteria is little more than an historical curiosity which owes more to neurology than to psychiatry or psychology; it does not refer to any specific syndrome, and its use generally reflects little more than a conviction that the wide range of symptoms displayed by such patients have no physical or medical foundation. Slater suggested that both on theoretical as well as on practical grounds the term should be avoided, since it is little more than a disguise for ignorance. Guze (1975), on the other hand, has argued strongly in favour of a system of classification based upon the medical model in which hysteria (Briquet's syndrome) is seen as a valid clinical entity which follows a predictable course.

Descriptions of hysteria still occasionally appear in the literature, as in Moss and McEvedy's (1966) paper on an epidemic of overbreathing which affected a group of 550 English schoolchildren. The authors relate this to personality factors, the affected children being described as high scorers on Eysenck's Neuroticism and Extraversion factors. Among the other recent reports of hysteria is that of Claridge (1967), who pointed to the higher incidence of hysterical symptoms, including even gross conversion reactions, among military populations. Claridge's explanation is also heavily reliant upon a physiologically based theory of personality.

Another personality theory of hysteria, albeit of a very different type, is the Freudian account. This has had a powerful influence upon psychiatry, as can be seen in the nosological systems currently in use (see Chap. 2). At the same time, it is unlikely that more than a minority of psychiatrists or psychologists would accept the details of Freudian theory whereby libidinal energy is converted into somatic disturbance. In the end, even Freud accepted that his account was unsatisfactory. 'One really does not know much that can be said about these symptoms . . . what the course is of the particular obscurity which surrounds symptom formation in conversion hysteria we are unable to guess' (Freud 1936). Nonetheless, this Freudian explanation of hysteria, whatever its defects, is more than Slater's diagnosis by exclusion.

One consequence of the Freudian view is that hysterical symptoms are frequently interpreted as a symbolic form of communication. Szasz (1961) has suggested that the hysterical patient is merely using the language of illness (albeit in an inappropriate way) to communicate with potential helpers. This sort of view led to an explanation of the high incidence of hysteria among military populations, which is entirely different from the physiological and medical accounts. Rabkin (1964) suggested that the conversion symptoms shown by army recruits reflect a fundamental disagreement between the doctor and patient about the nature of the patient's problems. When the civilian approaches his physician, he may describe his problem either in medical terms or in terms of his problems of living. In the army, Rabkin argues that the nature of the doctor-patient relationship is fundamentally different, and that this changed relationship encourages the development of hysterical disorders as a means of coping with the stresses of army life.

Unlike fullblown hysterical reactions (such as gross conversion symptoms), which seem to be comparatively rare, excessive concern about one's health or bodily functions is a rather more common problem. In general, it is also less likely to incapacitate the individual. However, in recent years there has been a reluctance to use the diagnosis of hypochondriacal neurosis, even in more severe cases. Although this category is contained in the European and American nosological systems ISD-8 and DSM II, such hypochondriacal concern is more often regarded as a manifestation of another more general anxiety disorder or of some personality trait.

Depressive reactions are one of the most common problems in the general population. Because of this, it is surprising that they have received so much less research attention than the neuroses characterised by anxiety and avoidance behaviours. Depression remains one of the more problematic disorders, and there is still considerable disagreement even over such basic issues as whether or not we should distinguish between neurotic and psychotic forms of depression (though there is considerable evidence to support such a distinction). There is further doubt about whether this distinction is equivalent to that between reactive and endogenous depression, or whether the two supposedly distinct sorts of disorder differ only in the severity of their symptoms (as the classical psycho-analysts maintain). The issue is confused even more by other workers who prefer to distinguish between primary and secondary depression or between agitated and retarded depressive states. Apart from their theoretical significance, such issues affect the ways in which the clinician approaches the problems being presented by the patient, and frequently they have direct implications for treatment. Patients diagnosed as neurotic or reactive depressives, for instance, do not usually respond well to ECT, and the presence of such other neurotic features as hypochondriasis, emotional lability and neurotic traits also seems to be associated with a poor response to 'medical' interventions of this sort (Mendels 1965; Carney et al. 1965).

As a research topic, depression seems to have had a particular attraction for cognitive theorists. Beck and Seligman each proposed cognitive accounts of depression which are interesting in their own right and which have also been useful in helping to correct the traditional psychiatric view of depression as a primary affective disorder. Beck (1967), for instance, suggested that the disturbances of the depressive patient can be seen in terms of three major cognitive patterns that lead the person to view himself, his world and his future in an idiosyncratic manner. The individual who has incorporated patterns of negative expectation is predisposed towards a depressive disorder, and when exposed to certain sorts of stressful events and experiences is more likely to become clinically depressed. As the primary triad of negative expectations become progressively more dominant, such cognitions lead to the other phenomena that are associated with the depressed state (depressed mood, suicidal wishes, behavioural inertia, etc.). The affective responses are therefore determined by the ways in which the individual structures his experiences.

This is broadly similar to Seligman's notion of learned helplessness as the crucial determinant of depression, though Seligman's account relies more heavily upon experimental evidence and upon the formulations of learning theory. Seligman noted that it is an essential feature of Pavlovian conditioning that the subject is helpless to control the outcome of his own responses. Overmier and Seligman (1967), for instance, showed that exposure to inescapable shock leads to escape/avoidance learning deficits. Seligman's theory suggests that the subject acquires the expectation that their responses and the outcome of their responses are independent. When the uncontrollable outcome is also traumatic, this produces increased anxiety followed by depression.

There are a number of difficulties with this account, both conceptual and empirical, but it remains a stimulating view of depression and has encouraged a considerable amount of research into this disorder. One of the alternative accounts to the cognitive emphasis of the learned helplessness model is that endogenous noradrenaline is differentially affected under conditions of controllable and uncontrollable shock (Weiss et al. 1976). Physiological and psycho-physiological studies have also contributed to our understanding of the mechanisms of the other neurotic disorders. Lader's (1967) results differentiated between different diagnostic groups of neurotic patients in terms of physiological measures. Patients with specific phobias, for instance, were differentiated from patients with other affective disorders, and it has been suggested both by Lader (1967) and by Kelly and Walter (1968) that phobic patients bear a closer ressemblance to normal groups than to other neurotic patients in terms of their physiological responses. Results of this sort also argue against a too-ready acceptance of the reclassification of DSM III in which the phobic disorders are defined as anxiety disorders. As a result they are included in the same category as panic attacks which are characterised by intense and widespread autonomic arousal, and with more chronic, generalised anxiety disorders in which motor tension and autonomic hyperactivity are defining characteristics. In the study of Kelly and Walter (1968), on the other hand, patients with phobic disorders differed from chronically anxious patients on almost every physiological measure that was used in the investigation.

There is always a temptation at this point to reach some conclusion to the effect that the best of each of the theories might be combined to produce a single comprehensive theory which would be more powerful than any of its components. There are, unfortunately, several objections which prevent the realisation of this pious hope. In the first place, the theories are often stated in such imprecise terms that it is difficult to see at which points they are in agreement and at which other points they make different predictions. For this reason alone it would be difficult to attempt any true synthesis. A further difficulty arises from the way in which the different accounts provide a general orientation or perspective upon the phenomena in which we are interested. Each theory operates as a selective filter upon our approach to the problem. An unfortunate complication of this has been the tendency for certain psychologists to display a sort of theoretical imperialism. Psychologists who work in medical settings will probably recognise this in the over-enthusiasm which some physicians display in their attempt to define social and psychological problems in medical terms. This same tendency is seen in those psychologists who are committed so completely to a particular theoretical perspective that they not only exclude alternative explanations of the neuroses, but that they also exclude alternative formulations of the problem. This results in disagreements of the most elusive kind – in which the proponents of different theories are unable to agree even upon such fundamental issues as what is to be explained. What a psycho-analyst understands by a neurosis may have little in common with what a conditioning theorist understands by the same term.

At present, no single theory has achieved general acceptance, and none can legitimately claim to offer a satisfactory explanation of each of the neurotic disorders (as contained in the psychiatric nosologies). There is a tendency for psychologists to be defensive about this lack of any agreed theory of neurosis. Such theoretical diversity need not, however, be regarded as a failure. Controversy may be the result of a lack of empirical information about a particular topic, and it may therefore have the useful function of stimulating research. It may also lead to a clarification of issues through the way in which the criticisms of opposing theories expose the assumptions underlying a particular theoretical approach. On the other hand, controversy can lead to a hardening of positions through the emotional heat generated in the course of debate: theoretical disputes can often produce a polarisation of views in which the various protagonists are forced into extreme positions that they do not really hold. A further danger is that definitions of a problem can be restricted in such a way as to fit the theory more exactly.

But whatever the disadvantages of controversy, it is unlikely that any theoretical resolution will take place in the near future. In an area of this sort where our present level of understanding is still rudimentary, provided that each of the theories pays attention to its own weaknesses as well as to the strengths of its rivals, it may ultimately be more productive to tolerate or even to encourage controversy than to enforce some premature synthesis.

10. References

Abramson LY, Seligman MEP, Teasdale JD (1978) Learned helplessness in humans: critique and reformulation. J Abnorm Psychol 87: 49–74

Adcock CJ (1965) A comparison of the concepts of Cattell and Eysenck. Br J Educ Psychol 35: 90–97

Adelman HM, Maatsch JL (1956) Learning and extinction based upon frustration, food reward, and exploratory tendency. J Exp Psychol 52: 311–315

Adelman MR (1977) A comparison of professionally employed lesbians and heterosexual women on the MMPI. Abnorm Sex Behav 6: 193–201

Adler A (1918) The neurotic constitution. Kegan Paul & Trench Trubner, New York

Adler A (1946) The practice and theory of individual psychology. Kegan Paul & Trench Trubner, London

Ajzen I, Fishbein M (1977) Attitude – behaviour relations: a theoretical analysis and review of empirical research. Psychol Bull 84: 888–928

Albee GW (1969) Emerging concepts of mental illness and models of treatment: the psychological point of view. Am J Psychiatry 125: 870–76

Amsel A (1962) Frustrative nonreward in partial reinforcement and discrimination learning: some recent history and a theoretical extension. Psychol Rev 69: 306–328

Argyle M, Trower P, Bryant B (1974) Explorations in the treatment of personality disorders and neuroses by social skills training. Br J Med Psychol 47: 63–72

Argyle M (1969) Social interaction. Methuen, London

Ash P (1949) The reliability of psychiatric diagnoses. J Abnorm Soc Psychol 44: 272–276

Azrin NH, Holz WC (1966) Punishment. In: Konig WK (ed) Operant behaviour: areas of research and application. Appleton-Century-Crofts, New York

Bandura A (1965) Influence of models reinforcement contingencies on the acquisition of imitative responses. J Pers Soc Psychol 1: 589–595

Bandura A (1969) Principles of behaviour modification. Holt, Rinehart & Winston, New York

Bandura A (1971) Psychological modelling: conflicting theories. Aldine & Atherton, Chicago

Bandura A (1974) Behaviour theory and the models of man. Am Psychol 29: 859–869

Bandura A (1977) Social learning theory. Prentice-Hall, Englewood Cliffs, NJ

Bandura A, Rosenthal TL (1966) Vicarious classical conditioning as a function of arousal level. J Pers Soc Psychol 3: 54–62

Bandura A, Grusec JE, Menlove FL (1967) Vicarious extinction of avoidance behaviour. J Pers Soc Psychol 5: 16–23

Barton WE (1959) Viewpoint of a clinician. In: Jahoda M (ed) Current concepts of positive mental health. Basic Books, New York

Beard GM (1869) Neurasthenia or nervous exhaustion. Boston Med Surg J 3: 159–271

Beck AT (1962) Reliability of psychiatric diagnoses: 1. a critique of systematic studies. Am J Psychiatry 119: 210–216

Beck AT (1967) Depression: clinical, experimental and theoretical aspects. Harper & Row, New York

Beck AT (1971) Cognition, affect and psychopathology. Arch Gen Psychiatry 24: 495–500

Beech HR, Watts F, Poole AD (1971) Classical conditioning of a sexual deviation: a preliminary note. Behav Ther 2: 400–402

Beech HR, Perigault J (1974) Toward a theory of obsessional disorder. In: Beech HR (ed) Obsessional states. Methuen, London

Bellak L, Hurvich M, Gediman HK (1973) Ego functions in schizophrenics, neurotics, and normals. Wiley, New York

Bem DJ, Allen A (1974) On predicting some of the people some of the time: the search for cross-situational consistences in behaviour. Psychol Rev 81: 506–520

Benjamin S, Marks IM, Huson J (1972) Active muscular relaxation in desensitisation of phobic patients. Psychol Med 2: 381–390

Berger SM (1962) Conditioning through vicarious instigation. Psychol Rev 69: 450–466

Berkley HJ (1901) A treatise on mental diseases. Kimpton, London

Berlyne DE (1954) Knowledge and stimulus-response psychology. Psychol Rev 61: 245

Blanchard EB, Hersen M (1976) Behavioural treatment of hysterical neurosis: symptom substitution and symptom return reconsidered. Psychiatry 39: 118–129

Block JD (1967) Monozygotic twin similarity in multiple psychophysiologic parameters and measures. In: Wortis J (ed) Recent advances in biological psychiatry, vol 9. Plenum Press, New York

Blum GS (1966) Psychodynamics: the science of unconscious mental forces. Wadsworth, Belmont, Ca.

Blumberg HH, Cohen SD, Dronfield BE, Mordecai EA, Roberts JC, Hawks D (1974) British opiate users I. People approaching London drug treatment centres. Int J Addict 9: 1–23

Bockoven JS (1956) Moral treatment in American psychiatry. J Nerv Ment Dis 3: 124, 167–194, 292–321

Bockoven JS (1963) Moral treatment in American psychiatry. Springer, Vienna, New York

Bolles RC, Grossen NE (1969) Effects of an informational stimulus on the acquisition of avoidance behaviour in rats. J comp physiol psychol 68: 90–99

Bolles RC (1970) Species-specific defence reactions and avoidance learning. Psychol Rev 77: 32–48

Borkovec TD (1976) Physiological and cognitive processes in the regulation of anxiety. In: Schwartz GE, Shapiro D (eds) Consciousness and self-regulation, vol 1. Plenum, New York

Boulougouris JC, Marks IM, Marset P (1971) Superiority of flooding (implosion) of desensitisation for reducing pathological fear. Behav Res Ther 9: 7–16

Brady JV, Porter RW, Conrad DG, Mason JW (1958) Avoidance behaviour and the development of gastroduodenal ulcers. J Exp Anal Behav 1: 69–72

Braginsky DD, Braginsky BM (1974) Mainstream psychology. A critique. Holt, Rinehart & Winston, New York

Bregman E (1934) An attempt to rectify the emotional attitudes of infants by the conditioned response technique. J Genet Psychol 45: 169–198

Breuer J, Freud S (1895) Studies on hysteria. Standard edition of the complete works of Sigmund Freud, vol II. Hogarth, London

Brewer WF (1974) There is no convincing evidence for operant or classical conditioning in adult humans. In: Weimer WB, Palermo DS (eds) Cognition and the symbolic processes. Wiley, New York

Brill AA (1936) Translator's introduction to C. G. Jung. The psychology of dementia praecox. Nerv Ment Dis Publishing Co., New York

Brill H (1967) Classification in psychiatry. In: Freedman AM, Kaplan HI (eds) Comprehensive textbook of psychiatry. Williams & Wilkins, Baltimore

Brill H (1974) Classification and nomenclature of psychiatric conditions. In: Arieti S (ed) American handbook of psychiatry, vol I. Basic Books, New York

Britton RS (1969) Psychiatric disorders in the mothers of disturbed children. J Child Psychol Psychiatry 10: 245

Broadhurst PL (1978) Drugs and the inheritance of behaviour. Plenum, London

Brown FW (1942) Heredity in the psychoneuroses. Proc R Soc Med 35: 785–790

Brown GW, Harris T (1978) Social origins of depression. Tavistock, London

Brown RT, Wagner AR (1964) Resistance to punishment and extinction following training with shock or nonreinforcement. J Exp Psychol 68: 503–507

Buchwald AM, Coyne JC, Cole CSA (1978) A critical evaluation of the learned helplessness model of depression. J Abnorm Psychol 87: 180–193

Burt C (1954) The assessment of personality. J Ment Sci 100, 1–28

Carney MWP, Roth M, Garside RF (1965) The diagnosis of depressive syndromes and the prediction of ECT response. Br J Psychiatry 111: 659–674

Caspari EW (1967) Behavioural consequences of genetic polymorphism in man: a summary. In: Genetic diversity and human behaviour. Spuhler JN (ed) Wenner-Gren Foundation Inc

Cattell RB (1946) Description and measurement of personality. World Books, New York

Cattell RB (1950) Personality: a systematic theoretical and factual study. McGraw-Hill, New York

Cattell RB (1952) Factor analysis. Greenwood, Westport

Cattell RB (1957a) Personality and motivation structure and measurement. World Books, New York

Cattell RB (1957b) The conceptual and test distinction of neuroticism and anxiety. J Clin Psychol 13: 221–233

Cattell RB, Kline P (1977) The scientific analysis of personality and motivation. Academic Press, New York

Cattell RB, Scheier IH (1961) Neuroticism and anxiety. Ronald, New York

Caveny EL, Wittson CL, Hunt WA, Herrman RS (1955) Psychiatric diagnosis, its nature and function. J Nerv Ment Dis 121: 367–373

Chesser ES (1976) Behaviour therapy: recent trends and current practice. Br J Psychiatry 129: 289–307

Church RM (1959) Emotional reactions of rats to the pain of others. J Comp Physiol Psychol 52: 132–134

Clare A (1976) Psychiatry in dissent. Tavistock, London

Claridge GS (1960) The excitation-inhibition balance in neurotics. In: Eysenck HJ (ed) Experiments in personality. Routledge & Kegan Paul, London

Claridge GS (1967) Personality and arousal. Pergamon, Oxford

Coates DB, Moyer S, Wellman B (1969) Yorklea study: symptoms, problems and life events. Can J Public Health 60: 471–481

Coates D, Moyer S, Wellman B (1969) The Yorklea study of urban mental health: symptoms, problems and life events. In: Boydell C, Grindstaff C, Whitehead P (eds) Deviant behaviour and societal reaction. Holt, Rinehart & Winston, Toronto

Coates DB, Moyer S, Kendall L, Howat MG (1976) Life-event changes and mental health. In: Sarason IG, Spielberger CD (eds) Stress and anxiety, vol 3. Wiley, New York

Cole S, Lejeune R (1972) Illness and the legitimation of failure. Am Sociol Rev 37: 347–356

Cook SW, Harris RE (1937) Verbal conditioning of the galvanic skin response. J Exp Psychol 21: 202–210

Costello CG (1970) Classification and psychopathology. In: Costello CG (ed) Symptoms of psychopathology. Wiley, New York

Cottrell NB, Wack DL, Sekerak GJ, Rittle RH (1968) Social facilitation of dominant responses by the presence of an audience and the mere presence of others. J Pers Soc Psychol 9: 245–250

Craighead WE, Kazdin AE, Mahoney M (1976) Behaviour modification, Houghton Mifflin, Boston, Ma.

Cullen W (1781) First lines on the practice of physic, vol 2. Creech, Edinburgh

Culpin M (1962) The conception of nervous disorder. Br J Med Psychol 35: 73–80

Curran D, Partridge M, Storey P (1972) Psychological medicine: an introduction to psychiatry. Churchill Livingstone, Edinburgh London

D'Amato MR, Schiff J (1964) Long-term discriminated avoidance performance in the rat. J Comp Physiol Psychol 57: 123–126

Davis JF, Malmo RB, Shagass C (1954) Electromyographic reaction to strong auditory stimulation in psychiatric patients. Can J Psychol 8: 177–186

Denker R (1946) Results of the treatment of psychoneuroses by the general practitioner. NJ State J Med 46: 2164–2166

Derogatis LR, Lipman RS, Covi L, Rickels K, Uhlenhuth EH (1970) Dimensions of outpatient neurotic pathology: a comparison of clinical versus an empirical assessment. J Consult Clin Psychol 34: 164–171

Derogatis LR, Covi L, Lipman RS, Davis DM, Rickels K (1971a) Social class and race as mediator variables in neurotic symptomatology. Arch Gen Psychiatry 25: 31–40

Derogatis LR, Lipman RS, Covi L, Rickels K (1971b) Neurotic symptom dimensions. Arch Gen Psychiatry 24: 454–464

Deutsch H (1944) Psychology of women. Grune & Stratton, New York, London

Dietz PE (1977) Social discrediting of psychiatry: the protasis of legal disenfranchisement. Am J Psychiatry 134: 1356–1360

Dollard J, Miller NE (1950) Personality and psychotherapy. McGraw-Hill, New York

DSM II (1968) Diagnostic and statistical manual of mental disorders, 2nd edn. Am Psychiatr Assoc, Washington, D.C.

DSM III (1978) Diagnostic and statistical manual of mental disorders, 3rd edn. Am Psychiatr Assoc, Washington, D.C.

DSM III (1978) Draft of the diagnostic and statistical manual of mental disorders. Third edition. Am Psychiatr Assoc, Washington

Ducey C, Simon B (1975) Ancient Greece and Rome. In: Howells JG (ed) World history of psychiatry. Bailliere Tindall, London

Eiser JR (1979) Addiction as attribution. Paper presented to European Association of Experimental Social Psychology, Cumbria, England

Eiser JR (1978) Interpersonal attribution. In: Tajfel H, Fraser C (eds) Introducing social psychology. Penguin Books, New York

Eiser JR (1979) Addiction as attribution. In: Eiser JR (ed) Social psychology and behavioural medicine. Wiley, London

Ellenberger HF (1970) The discovery of the unconscious. Allen Lane, London

Ellenberger HF (1974) Psychiatry from ancient to modern times. In: Arieti S (ed) American handbook of psychiatry. Basic Books, New York, vol I.

Ellis A (1962) Reason and emotion in psychotherapy. Lyle Stuart, New York

Endler NS, Hunt J McV (1966) Sources of behavioural variance as measured by the S-R inventory of anxiousness. Psychol Bull 65: 336–346

Endler NS, Hunt J McV (1969) Generalisability of contributions from sources of variance in the S-R inventories of anxiousness. J Pers 37: 1–20

Engel GL (1972) Is psychiatry failing in its responsibility to medicine? Am J Psychiatry 128: 1561–1563

Erikson K (1957) Patient role and social uncertainty: a dilemma of the mentally ill. Psychiatry 20: 263–274

Essen-Möller E (1956) Individual traits and morbidity in a Swedish rural population. Acta Psychiatr Scand [Suppl] 100

Essen-Möller E (1967) On classification of mental disorders. Acta Psychiatr Scand 37: 119–126

Everitt BS, Gourlay AJ, Kendall RE (1971) An attempt at validation of traditional psychiatric syndromes by cluster analysis. Br J Psychiatry 119: 399–412

Eysenck HJ (1947a) Dimensions of personality. Routledge & Kegan Paul, London

Eysenck HJ (1947b) Screening out the neurotic. Lancet 1: 530

Eysenck HJ (1955) Psychiatric diagnosis as a psychological and statistical problem. Psychol Rep 1: 3–17

Eysenck HJ (1957) The dynamics of anxiety and hysteria. Routledge & Kegan Paul, London

Eysenck HJ (1959) Learning theory and behaviour therapy. J Ment Sci 105: 61–75

Eysenck HJ (1960a) Modern learning theory. In: Eysenck HJ (ed) Behaviour therapy and the neuroses. Pergamon, London

Eysenck HJ (1960b) Symposium: the development of moral values in children. Br J Educ Psychol 30: 11–21

Eysenck HJ (1960c) A rational system of diagnosis and therapy in mental illness. In: Progress in clinical psychology, vol IV. Grune & Stratton, New York, London

Eysenck HJ (1961) Classification and the problem of diagnosis. In: Eysenck HJ (ed) Handbook of abnormal psychology. Basic Books, New York

Eysenck HJ, Claridge G (1962) The position of hysterics and dysthymics in a two-dimensional framework of personality description. J abnorm soc psychol 69: 46–55

Eysenck HJ (1965) Extraversion and the acquisition of eyeblink and GSR conditioned responses. Psychol Bull 63: 258–270

Eysenck HJ (1967) The biological basis of personality. Thomas, Springfield, Ill.

Eysenck HJ (1968) A theory of the incubation of anxiety/fear responses. Behav Res Ther 6: 309–321

Eysenck HJ (1970a) The classification of depressive illness. Br J Psychiatry 117: 241–250

Eysenck HJ (1970b) The structure of human personality. Methuen, London

Eysenck HJ (1972a) Primaries or second-order factors: a critical consideration of Cattell's 16PF battery. Br J Soc Clin Psychol 11: 265–269

Eysenck HJ (1972b) Traits. In: Eysenck HJ, Meili WAR (eds) Encyclopedia of psychology, vol 3. Search, London

Eysenck HJ (1975a) The future of psychiatry. Methuen, London

Eysenck HJ (1975b) Anxiety and the natural history of neurosis. In: Spielberger C, Sarason I (eds) Stress and anxiety, vol 1. Hemisphere, New York

Eysenck HJ (1976) The learning theory model of neurosis – a new approach. Behav Res Ther 14: 251–267

Eysenck HJ (1977) Crime and personality. Routledge & Kegan Paul, London

Eysenck HJ (1979) The conditioning model of neurosis. In: Behavioural and brain science, 2: 155–199

Eysenck HJ, Eysenck SBG (1969) Personality structure and measurement. Routledge & Kegan Paul, London

Eysenck HJ, Eysenck SBG (1975) Manual of the Eysenck personality questionnaire. Hodder & Stoughton, London

Eysenck HJ, Rachman S (1965) The causes and cures of neurosis. Routledge & Kegan Paul, London

Eysenck SBG (1956) Neurosis and psychosis: an experimental analysis. J Ment Sci 102: 517–529

Fahrenberg J (1977) Physiological concepts in personality research. In: Cattell RB, Dreger RM (eds) Handbook of modern personality theory. Wiley, New York

Farrell BA (1951) The scientific testing of psychoanalytic findings and theory. Br J Med Psychol 24: 35–51

Farrell BA (1961) On the character of psychoanalytic discourse. Br J Med Psychol 34: 7–21

Farrell BA (1967) The criteria for a psychoanalytic interpretation. In: Gustafson DF (ed) Essays in philosophical psychology. Macmillan, London

Feldman MP (1966) Aversion therapy for sexual deviations: a critical review. Psychol Bull 65: 65–69

Feldman MP, MacCulloch MJ (1971) Homosexual behaviour: therapy and assessment. Pergamon, Oxford

Fenischel O (1945) The psychoanalytic theory of neurosis. Norton, New York

Fenton N (1926) Shell shock and its aftermath. Mosby, St. Louis

Flew A (1978) Mental disease. J Med Ethics 4: 89–90

Foulds GA (1955) The reliability of psychiatric, and the validity of psychological diagnoses. J Ment Sci 101: 851–862

Foulds GA, Bedford A (1975) Hierarchy of classes of personal illness. Psychol Med 5: 181–192

Foulds GA, Bedford A (1976) The relationship between anxiety-depression and the neuroses. Br J Psychiatry 128: 166–168

Frank G (1975) Psychiatric diagnosis: a review of research. Pergamon, New York

Freud S (1893–1895) Studies on hysteria. Standard edition of the complete works of Sigmund Freud, vol II. Hogarth, London

Freud S (1893–1899) Early psychoanalytic publications. Standard edition of the complete works of Sigmund Freud, vol III. Hogarth, London

Freud S (1900) The interpretation of dreams. Allen & Unwin, London

901–1905) A case of hysteria, three essays on sexuality and other works. Standard edition of the complete works of Sigmund Freud, vol VII. Hogarth, London

Freud S (1905) Three essays on the theory of sexuality. Basic Books, New York

Freud S (1906–1908) Jensen's 'Gravida', Standard edition of the complete works of Sigmund Freud, vol IX. Hogarth, London

Freud S (1909) The cases of 'Little Hans' and the 'Rat Man'. Standard edition of the complete works of Sigmund Freud, vol X. Hogarth, London

Freud S (1911–1913) Case history of Schreber, papers on technique. Standard edition of the complete works of Sigmund Freud, vol XII. Hogarth, London

Freud S (1914–1916) A history of the psychoanalytic movement, papers on metapsychology and other works. Standard edition of the complete works of Sigmund Freud, vol XIV. Hogarth, London

Freud S (1Freud S (1917) Introductory lectures on psycho-analysis. Standard edition of the com-
    plete works of Sigmund Freud, vol XVI. Hogarth, London
Freud S (1923–1925) The ego and the id and other works. Standard edition of the complete works
    of Sigmund Freud, vol XIX. Hogarth, London
Freud S (1924) Collected papers, vol II. Hogarth, London
Freud S (1925–1926) An autobiographical study, inhibitions symptoms and anxiety, lay analysis and
    other works. Standard edition of the complete works of Sigmund Freud, vol XX. Hogarth,
    London
Freud S (1932–1936) New introductory lectures. Standard edition of the complete works of Sig-
    mund Freud, vol XXII. Hogarth, London
Freud S (1936) The problem of anxiety. Norton, New York
Freud S (1937–1939) Moses and monotheism, an outline of psychoanalysis and other works. Stand-
    ard edition of the complete works of Sigmund Freud, vol XXIII. Hogarth, London
Frith CD, Johnstone EC, Owens D, McPherson K (1978) The phenomenological, pharmacological
    and psychophysiological characteristics of neurotic outpatients to whom no diagnosis has been
    applied. Proc 11th C.I.N.P. Conference, Vienna
Frolov YP (1938) Pavlov and his school. Kegan Paul, London
Fromm E (1960) The fear of freedom. Routledge & Kegan Paul, London
Garcia J, Koelling R (1966) Relation of cue to consequence in avoidance learning. Psychosom Sci 4:
    123–124
Garmany G (1958) Depressive states: their aetiology and treatment. Br Med J 2: 341–344
Giorgi A (1970) Psychology as a human science. Harper & Row, New York
Glass, DC, Singer JE (1972) Urban stress: experiments on noise and urban stressors. Academic
    Press, New York
Gleitman H, Nachmias J, Neisser U (1954) The S-R reinforcement theory of extinction. Psychol
    Rev 61: 23–33
Goffman E (1961) Asylums: essays on the social situation of mental patients and other inmates.
    Anchor, New York
Goldberg DP (1972) The detection of psychiatric illness by questionnaire. Maudsley Monographs.
    Oxford University Press, London
Goldstein IB (1964) Physiological responses in anxious women patients. A study of autonomic
    activity and muscle tension. Arch Gen Psychiatry 10: 382–388
Gormezano I, Moore JW (1969) Classical conditioning. In: Marx MM (ed) Learning processes.
    Macmillan, London
Gossop MR (1974) Movement variables and the subsequent following response of the domestic
    chick. Anim Behav 22: 982–986
Gossop MR (1978a) A comparative study of oral and intravenous drug dependent patients on three
    dimensions of personality. Int J Addict 13: 135–142
Gossop MR (1978b) Drug dependence, crime and personality among female addicts. Drug Alcohol
    Depend 3: 359–364
Gossop MR (1978c) Drug dependence: a study of the relationship between motivational, cognitive,
    social and historical factors, and treatment variables. J Nerv Ment Dis 166: 44–50
Gossop MR (1979) Drug dependence: a reappraisal. In: Oborne DJ, Gruneberg MM, Eiser JR
    (eds) Research in psychology and medicine, vol 2. Academic Press, London
Gossop MR, Connell PH (1975) Attitudes of oral and intravenous multiple drug users toward drugs
    of abuse. Int J Addict 10: 459–472
Gossop MR, Kristjansson I (1977) Crime and personality: a comparison of convicted and non-
    convicted drug dependent males. Br J Criminol 17: 264–273
Gottesman II (1963) Heritability of personality: a demonstration. Psychol Monogr 77/9
Gough HG (1946) Diagnostic patterns on the MMPI. J Clin Psychol 2: 23–37
Gove WR (1970) Societal reaction as an explanation of mental illness: an evaluation. Am Sociol
    Rev 35: 873–884
Gove WR (1975) Labelling and mental illness: a critique. In: Gove WR (ed) The labelling of
    deviance. Wiley, London
Gove WR, Fain T (1973) The stigma of mental hospitalisation. Arch Gen Psychiatry 28: 494–500
Gove WR, Howell P (1974) Individual resources and mental hospitalisation: a comparison and
    evaluation of the societal reaction and psychiatric perspectives. Am Sociol Rev 39: 86–100

Grant DA (1964) Classical and operant conditioning. In: Melton AW (ed) Categories of human learning. Academic Press, New York

Gray J (1970a) Sodium amobarbital, the hippocampal theta rhythm and the partial reinforcement extinction effect. Psychol Rev 77: 465–480

Gray J (1970b) The psychophysiological basis of introversion-extraversion. Behav Res Ther 8: 249–266

Gray J (1971) The psychology of fear and stress. World University Library, London

Gray JA (1972) The psychophysiological basis of introversion-extraversion: a modification of Eysenck's theory. In: Biological bases of individual behaviour. Nebylitsyn VD & Gray JA (eds) Academic Press, New York

Gray J (1973) Causal theories of personality and how to test them. In: Royce JR (ed) Multivariate analysis and psychological theory. Academic Press, London

Gray JA (1975) Elements of a two-process theory of learning. Academic Press, London

Gray JA (1976) The neuropsychology of anxiety. In: Sarason IG, Spielberger CD (eds) Stress and anxiety, vol 3. Wiley, New York

Greenson RR (1967) The technique and practice of psychoanalysis. International University Press, New York

Griesinger W (1876) Die Pathologie und Therapie der psychischen Krankheiten. Wreden, Brunswik

Grinker RR, Miller J, Sabshin M, Nunn R, Nunally JC (1961) The phenomena of depressions. Harper & Row, New York

Guilford JP, Guilford RB (1934) An analysis of the factors in a typical test of introversion-extroversion. J Abnorm Soc Psychol 28: 377–399

Guilford JP, Guilford RB (1936) Personality factors S, E, and M, and their measurement. J Psychol 2: 109–127

Guilford JP, Zimmerman WS (1956) Fourteen dimensions of temperament. Psychol Monogr 70/10

Guthrie ER (1952) The psychology of learning. Harper, New York

Guze SB (1975) The validity and significance of the clinical diagnosis of hysteria (Briquet's syndrome). Am J Psychiatry 132: 138–141

Hagnell O (1959) Neuroses and other nervous disturbances in a population living in a rural area of Southern Sweden, investigated in 1947 and 1957. Acta Psychiatr Scand [Suppl] 136: 214–219

Hagnell O (1968) A Swedish epidemiological study: the Lundby project. Soc Psychiatry 3: 75–77

Hallam RS (1974) Extinction of ruminations: a case study. Behav Ther 5: 565–568

Hallam RS, Rachman S (1972) Some effects of aversion therapy on patients with sexual disorders. Behav Res Ther 10: 171–180

Hallam RS, Rachman S, Falkowski W (1972) Subjective, attitudinal and physiological effects of electrical aversion therapy. Behav Res Ther 10: 1–13

Hanusa BH, Schulz R (1977) Attributional mediators of learned helplessness. J Pers Soc Psychol 35: 602–611

Hartmann H (1960) Toward a concept of mental health. Br J Med Psychol 33: 243–248

Hartshorne H, May MA (1928) Studies in the nature of character, vol 1. Studies in deceit. Macmillan, New York

Hartshorne H, May MA, Shuttleworth FK (1929) Studies in the nature of character, vol 3. Studies in the organisation of character. Macmillan, New York

Harzem P, Miles TR (1978) Conceptual issues in operant psychology. Wiley, London

Hearst E (1969) Aversive conditioning and external stimulus control. In: Campbell BA, Church RM (eds) Punishment and aversive behaviour. Appleton-Century-Crofts, New York

Hebb DO (1947) Spontaneous neurosis in chimpanzees: theoretical relations with clinical and experimental phenomena. Psychosom Med 9: 3–16

Heilbrunn (1963) Results with psychoanalytic therapy. Am J Psychother 17: 427–435

Helmholtz H von (1866) Handbuch der physiologischen Optik. Hamburg, Leipzig

Hempel CG (1961) Introduction to the problems of taxonomy. In: Zubin J (ed) Field studies in the mental disorders. Grune & Stratton, New York, London

Henderson D, Batchelor IRC (1962) Textbook of psychiatry. Oxford University Press, London

Hendrick I (1958) Facts and theories of psychoanalysis. Dell, New York

Hersen M, Eisler RM (1976) Social skills training. In: Craighead WE, Kazdin AE, Mahoney MJ (eds) Behaviour modification. Houghton Mifflin, Boston

Hine FR, Williams RB (1975) Dimensional diagnosis and the medical student's grasp of psychiatry. Arch Gen Psychiatry 32: 525–528

Hodgson R, Rachman S, Marks I (1972) The treatment of chronic obsessive-compulsive neurosis: follow-up and further findings. Behav Res Ther 10: 181–189

Hoghughi MS, Forrest AR (1970) Eysenck's theory of criminality. Br J Criminol 10: 240–254

Hollingshead AB, Redlich FC (1958) Social class and mental illness: a community study. Wiley, New York

Holz WC, Azrin NH (1961) Discriminative properties of punishment. J Exp Anal Behav 4: 225–232

Horney K (1936) Culture and neurosis. Am Sociol Rev 1: 221–230

Horney K (1937) The neurotic personality of our time. Kegan Paul & Trench Trubner, London

Horney K (1946) Our inner conflicts. Kegan Paul & Trench Trubner, London

Howe ES (1958) GSR conditioning in anxiety states, normals and chronic functional schizophrenic subjects. J Abnorm Soc Psychol 56: 183–189

Howells JG (1970) Nosology of psychiatry. Society of Clinical Psychiatrists, Ipswich

Hull CL (1932) The goal gradient hypothesis and maze learning. Psychol Rev 39: 25–43

Hull CL (1937) Mind, mechanism, and adaptive behaviour. Psychol Rev 44: 1–32

Hull CL (1943) Principles of behaviour: an introduction to behaviour theory. Appleton-Century-Crofts, New York

Hull CL (1952) A behaviour system. Yale University Press, New Haven

Humphreys LG (1939) The effect of random alternation of reinforcement on the acquisition and extinction of conditioned eyelid reactions. J Exp Psychol 25: 141–158

Hunt HC (1932) A retired habituation. A history of The Retreat. York, Lewis, London

Hunt WA, Wittson CL, Hunt CB (1953) A theoretical and practical analysis of the diagnostic process. In: Hoch PH, Zubin J (eds) Current problems in psychiatric diagnosis. Grune & Stratton, New York, London

Hunter R (1973) Psychiatry and neurology: psychosyndrome or brain disease. Proc R Soc Med 66: 359–364

Hunter R, Macalpine I (1970) Three hundred years of psychiatry. 1535–1860. Oxford University Press, London

Ingham JG (1966) Changes in MPI scores in neurotic patients: a three year follow-up. Br J Psychiatry 112: 931–939

ICD-8 (1967) Manual of the international statistical classification of diseases, injuries, and causes of death. WHO, Geneva

Jacobsen CF, Wolfe JB, Jackson TA (1935) An experimental analysis of the frontal association areas in primates. J Nerv Ment Dis 82: 1–14

Jahoda M (1958) Current concepts of positive mental health. Basic Books, New York

Janet P (1891) Etude sur un cas d'aboulie et d'idées fixes. Rev Philos 31: 258–287, 382–407

Janet P (1895) J. M. Charcot, son oeuvre psychologique. Rev Philos 39: 569–604

Janet P (1909) Les névroses. Flammarion, Paris

Jaspers K (1972) General psychopathology, 4th edn. Manchester University Press, Manchester

Jellinek EM (1939) Some principles of psychiatric classification. Psychiatry 2: 161–165

Jones MC (1924) A laboratory study of fear. Pedagog Sem 31: 308–315

Jones E (1950) The concept of a normal mind. In: Halmos P, Iliffe A (eds) Philosophical Library, New York, Readings in general psychology.

Jones MC (1975) A 1924 pioneer looks at behaviour therapy. J Behav Ther Exp Psychiatry 6: 181–187

Kaelbling R, Volpe PA (1963) Constancy of psychiatric diagnoses in readmission. Compr Psychiatry 4: 29–39

Kagan J (1967) On the need for relativism. Am Psychol 22: 131–142

Kamiya J (1969) Operant control of the EEG rhythm and some of its reported effects on consciousness. In: Tart CT (ed) Altered states of consciousness. Wiley, New York

Kanfer FH, Saslow G (1967) Behavioural analysis: an alternative to diagnostic classification. In: Millon T (ed) Theories of psychopathology. Saunders, Philadelphia London

Kanfer FH, Phillips JS (1970) Learning foundations of behaviour therapy. Wiley, New York

Kaplan HI, Kaplan HS (1956) A historical survey of psychosomatic medicine. J Nerv Ment Dis 124: 546–568

Katz A, Webb L, Stotland E (1971) Cognitive influences on the rate of GSR extinction. J Exp Res Pers 5: 208–215

Katz M, Cole JO, Lowery HA (1969) Studies of the diagnostic process: the influence of symbolic perception, past experience, and ethnic background on diagnostic decisions. Am J Psychiatry 125: 937–947

Kelley HH (1948) First impression in interpersonal relations. Cited in: Krech D, Crutchfield R, Ballachey E (eds) Individual in society. McGraw-Hill, New York

Kelley HH (1950) The warm-cold variable in first impressions of persons. J Pers 18: 431–439

Kelly DHW (1966) Measurement of anxiety by forearm blood flow. Br J Psychiatry 112: 789–798

Kelly DHW, Walter CJS (1968) The relationship between clinical diagnosis and anxiety, assessed by forearm blood flow and other measurements. Br J Psychiatry 114: 611–626

Kelly G (1955) The psychology of personal constructs. Norton, New York

Kendell RE (1975) The role of diagnosis in psychiatry. Blackwell, Oxford

Kiloh LG, Andrews G, Neilson M, Bianchi G (1972) The relationship of the syndromes called endogenous and neurotic depression. Br J Psychiatry 121: 183–196

Kiloh LG, Garside RF (1963) The independence of neurotic depression and endogenous depression. Br J Psychiat 109: 451–63

King LS (1958) The medical world of the eighteenth century. University of Chicago Press, Chicago

Klein M (1960) On mental health. Br J Med Psychol 33: 237–241

Kline P (1968) Obsessional traits, obsessional symptoms and anal eroticism. Br J Med Psychol 41: 299–305

Knight RP (1941) Evaluation of the results of psychoanalytic therapy. Am J Psychiatry 98: 434–446

Knoff WF (1970) A history of the concept of neurosis, with a memoir of William Cullen. Am J Psychiatry 127: 80–84

Kraeplin E (1896) Psychiatrie. Barth, Leipzig

Kraeplin E (1906) Lectures on clinical psychiatry. Bailliere Tindall, London

Kreitman N (1961) The reliability of psychiatric diagnosis. J Ment Sci 107: 876–886

Kreitman N, Sainsbury P, Morrissey J, Towers J, Scrivener J (1961) The reliability of psychiatric assessment: an analysis. J Ment Sci 107: 887–908

Kuhn TS (1970) Logic of discovery or psychology of research. In: Lakatos I, Musgrove A (eds) Criticism and the growth of knowledge. Cambridge University Press, Cambridge

Lader M (1967) Palmar skin conductance measures in anxiety and phobic states. J Psychosom Res 11: 271–281

Lader MH (1969) Psychophysiological aspects of anxiety. In: Lader MH (ed) Studies of anxiety. Headley, Kent

Lader MH, Gelder MG, Marks IM (1967) Palmar skin conductance measures as predictors of response to desensitisation. J Psychosom Res 11: 283–290

Lader MH, Noble P (1975) The affective disorders. In: Venables PH, Christie MJ (eds) Research in psychophysiology. Wiley, London

Lader MH, Wing L (1966) Psychophysiological measures, sedative drugs and morbid anxiety. Oxford University Press, London

Lakatos I (1970) Falsification and the methodology of scientific research programmes. In: Lakatos I, Musgrove A (eds) Criticism and the growth of knowledge. Cambridge University Press, Cambridge

Laplanche J, Pontalis JB (1973) The language of psychoanalysis. Hogarth, London

Laughlin HP (1967) The neuroses. Butterworths, Washington, D.C.

Lazare A (1973) Hidden conceptual models in clinical psychiatry. N Engl J Med 288: 345–351

Lazarus AA, Rachman S (1960) The use of systematic desensitisation psychotherapy. In: Eysenck HJ (ed) Behaviour therapy and the neuroses. Pergamon, Oxford

Lemert E (1967) Human deviance, social problems and social control. Prentice Hall, New Jersey

Lesse S (1970) Anxiety: its components, development and treatment. Grune & Stratton, New York, London

Levine M (1942) Psychotherapy in medical practice. Macmillan, New York

Levy R, Meyer V (1971) Ritual prevention in obsessional patients. Proc R Soc Med 64: 1115–1118

Lewin K (1935) A dynamic theory of personality. McGraw-Hill, New York

Lewinsohn PM, Mischel W, Chaplin W, Barton R (1980) Social competence and depression: the role of illusory self-perceptions. J Abnorm Psychol 89: 203–212

Lewis AJ (1934) Melancholia: a clinical survey of depressive states. J Ment Sci 80: 277–378
Lewis AJ (1951) Henry Maudsley: his work and influence. J Ment Sci 97: 255–277
Lewis AJ (1958) Between guesswork and certainty in psychiatry. Lancet 1: 170–175, 227–230
Liberman RP, Raskin DE (1971) Depression: a behavioural formulation. Arch Gen Psychiat 24: 515–523
Libet JM, Lewinsohn PM (1973) Concept of social skill with special reference to the behaviour of depressed persons. J Consult Clin Psychol 40: 304–312
Loevinger J (1955) Diagnosis and measurement: a reply to Eysenck. Psychol Rep 1: 277–278
Lorr M, O'Connor JP (1957) The relation between neurosis and psychosis: a re-analysis. J Ment Sci 103: 375–380
Lucas CJ, Kelvin RP, Ojha AB (1965) The psychological health of the preclinical medical student. Br J Psychiatry 111: 473–478
Ludwig AM (1975) The psychiatrist as physician. J Am Med Assoc 234: 603–604
Ludwig AM, Othner EO (1977) The medical basis of psychiatry. Am J Psychiatry 134: 1087–1092
Luria AR (1961) The role of speech in the regulation of normal and abnormal behaviour. Pergamon, New York
McGuire RJ, Mowbray RM, Vallance RC (1963) The Maudsley personality inventory used with psychiatric inpatients. Br J Psychol 54: 157–166
Mackay D (1975) Clinical psychology: theory and therapy. Methuen, London
Macmillan MB (1976) Beard's concept of neurasthenia and Freud's concept of the actual neuroses. J Hist Behav Sci 12: 376–390
Maher BA (1966) Principles of psychopathology. McGraw-Hill, New York
Mahoney M (1974) Cognition and behaviour modification. Ballinger, Cambridge
Mahoney MJ (1977) Reflections on the cognitive-learning trend in psychotherapy. Am Psychol 32: 5–13
Mahoney MJ, Kazdin AE, Lesswing NJ (1974) Behaviour modification: delusion or deliverance? In: Franks CM, Wilson GT (eds) Annual review of behaviour therapy and practice, vol 2. Brunner-Mazel, New York
Malmo RB (1957) Anxiety and behavioural arousal. Psych Rev 64: 276–87
Malmo RB, Shagass C (1952) Studies of blood pressure in psychiatric patients under stress. Psychosom Med 14: 82–93
Mapother E (1926) Manic-depressive psychosis. Br Med J 2: 872–879
Marks IM (1969) Fears and phobias. Heinemann, London
Marks IM (1970) The classification of phobic disorders. Br J Psychiatry 116: 377–386
Marks IM (1973a) Research in neurosis: a selective review. 1. Causes and courses. Psychol Med 3: 436–454
Marks IM (1973b) New approaches to the treatment of obsessive-compulsive disorders. J Nerv Ment Dis 156: 420–426
Marks IM (1974) Research in neurosis: a selective review. 2. Treatment. Psychol Med 4: 89–109
Marks IM, Gelder MG (1967) Transvestism and fetishism: clinical and psychological changes during faradic aversion. Br J Psychiatry 113: 711–729
Marks IM, Hodgson R, Rachman S (1975) Treatment of chronic obsessive-compulsive neurosis by in vivo exposure. Br J Psychiatry 127: 349–364
Marx MH, Hillix WA (1963) Systems and theories in psychology. McGraw-Hill, New York
Marzillier J (1978) Outcome studies of skills training: a review. In: Trower P, Bryant B, Argyle M (eds) Social skills and mental health. Methuen, London
Maslow AH, Mittelmann (1951) Principles of abnormal psychology. Harper, New York
Masserman JG, Carmichael HT (1938) Diagnosis and prognosis in psychiatry: with a follow-up study of the results of short-term general hospital therapy of psychiatric cases. J Ment Sci 84: 893–946
Masters WH, Johnson VE (1970) Human sexual inadequacy. Little, Brown, Boston
Mather MD (1970) The treatment of an obsessional-compulsive patient by discrimination learning and reinforcement of decision making. Behav Res Ther 8: 315–318
Maturana HR, Lettvin JY, McCulloch WS, Pitts WB (1960) Anatomy and physiology of vision in the frog. J Gen Physiol 43: 129–175
Maudsley H (1899) The pathology of mind. Appleton, New York
Meehl PE (1946) Profile analysis of the MMPI in differential diagnosis. J Appl Psychol 30: 517–524

Meehl PE (1973) Psychodiagnosis: selected papers. University of Minnesota Press, Minnesota

Meichenbaum D (1976) Toward a cognitive theory of self-control. In: Schwartz GE, Shapiro D (eds) Consciousness and self-regulation. Advances in research, vol 1. Plenum, New York

Meichenbaum D (1977) Cognitive-behaviour modification. Plenum, New York

Meichenbaum D, Cameron R (1974) The clinical potential of modifying what clients say to themselves. Psychother Theor Res Pract 11: 103–117

Melges FT, Bowlby J (1969) Types of helplessness in psychopathological process. Arch Gen Psychiatry 20: 690–699

Mendels J (1965) Electroconvulsive therapy and depression. 2. Significance of endogenous and reactive syndromes. Br J Psychiatry 111: 682–686

Mendelson M (1974) Psychoanalytic concepts of depression. Spectrum, New York

Menninger K (1948) Changing concepts of disease. Ann Intern Med 29: 318–325

Menninger K, Mayman M, Pruyser P (1963) The vital balance. Viking, New York

Meyer V, Chesser ES (1970) Behaviour therapy in clinical psychiatry. Penguin, Harmondsworth, Middx

Meyer V, Crisp AH (1970) Phobias. In: Costello CG (ed) Symptoms of psychopathology. Wiley, New York

Meyer V, Levy R (1970) Behaviour treatment of a homosexual with compulsive rituals. Br J Med Psychol 43: 63–67

Miles TR (1966) Eliminating the unconscious. Pergamon, Oxford

Miller NE (1948) Studies of fear as an acquirable drive. I. Fear as motivation and fear-reduction as reinforcement in the learning of new responses. J Exp Psychol 38: 89–101

Miller NE (1959) Liberalisation of basic S-R concepts: extensions to conflict behaviour, motivation, and social learning. In: Koch S (ed) Psychology: a study of a science, vol 2. McGraw-Hill, New York

Miller NE (1969) Learning of visceral and glandular responses. Science 163: 434–445

Mischel W (1968) Personality and assessment. Wiley, New York

Mischel W (1969) Continuity and change in personality. Am Psychol 24: 1012–1018

Mischel W (1973) Toward a cognitive social learning reconceptualisation of personality. Psychol Rev 80: 252–283

Mischel W (1977) On the future of personality measurement. Am Psychol 32: 246–254

Mischel W (1979) On the interface of cognition and personality: beyond the person-situation debate. Am Psychol 34: 740–754

Money-Kyrle RE (1957) Psychoanalysis and ethics. In: Klein M, Heimann P, Money-Kyrle RE (eds) New directions in psychoanalysis. Basic Books, New York

Monroe LJ (1967) Psychological and physiological differences between good and poor sleepers. J Abnorm Soc Psychol 72: 255–264

Mora G (1967) History of psychiatry. In: Freedman AM, Kaplan HI (eds) Comprehensive textbook of psychiatry. Williams & Wilkins, Baltimore

Moss P, McEvedy C (1966) An epidemic of overbreathing among schoolgirls. Br Med J 2: 1295–1300

Mowrer OH (1938) Enuresis: a method for its study and treatment. Am J Orthopsychiat 8: 436–459

Mowrer OH (1939) A stimulus-response analysis of anxiety and its role as a reinforcing agent. Psychol Rev 46: 553–565

Mowrer OH (1950) Learning theory and personality dynamics. Arnold, New York

Mowrer OH (1969) Psychoneurotic defences (including deception) as punishment-avoidance strategies. In: Campbell BA, Church RM (eds) Punishment and aversive behaviour. Appleton-Century-Crofts, New York

Mowrer OH (1976) Enuresis: the beginning work. Paper presented to Annual Convention of Am Psychol Assoc 1976, Washington, D.C.

Mowrer OH, Ullman AD (1945) Time as a determinant in integrative learning. Psychol Rev 52: 61–90

Muezinger KF (1934) Motivation in learning: I. electric shock for correct response in the visual discrimination habit. J Comp Physiol Psychol 17: 267–277

Munroe RL (1957) Schools of psychoanalytic thought. Hutchinson, London

Myerson A (1936) Neuroses and neuropsychoses. Am J Psychiatry 93: 263–301

Nagera H (1969) Basic psychoanalytic concepts on the libido theory. Allen & Unwin, London
Nebylitsyn VD (1964) An investigation of the connection between sensitivity and strength of the nervous system. In: Gray JA (ed) Pavlov's typology. Pergamon, London
Nichols KA (1974) Severe social anxiety. Br J Med Psychol 47: 301–306
Nisbett RE, Schachter S (1966) Cognitive manipulation of pain. J Exp Soc Psychol 2: 227–236
Nisbett RE, Valins S (1971) Perceiving the causes of one's own behaviour. In: Jones EE et al. (eds) Attribution: perceiving the causes of behaviour. General Learning Press, New Jersey
Norris V (1959) Mental illness in London. Chapman & Hall, London
O'Connor JP (1953) A statistical test of psychoneurotic syndromes. J Abnorm Soc Psychol 48: 581–584
Offer D, Sabshin M (1966) Normality. In: Freedman AM, Kaplan HI (eds) Comprehensive textbook of psychiatry. Williams & Wilkins, Baltimore
Offer D, Sabshin M (1974) The concept of normality. In: Arieti S (ed) The foundations of Psychiatry. Vol I. Basic Books, New York
Osgood CE (1953) Method and theory in experimental psychology. Oxford University Press, New York
Overmier JB, Seligman MEP (1967) Effects of inescapable shock on subsequent escape and avoidance learning. J Comp Physiol Psychol 63: 28–33
Parsons T (1952) The social system. Tavistock, London
Parsons T (1965) Social structure and personality. Collier Macmillan, London
Paul GL (1966) Insight versus desensitisation in psychotherapy: an experiment in anxiety reduction. Stanford University Press, Stanford, Ca.
Pavlov IP (1927) Conditioned reflexes. Oxford University Press, London
Pavlov IP (1928) Lectures on conditioned reflexes, vol 1. International, New York
Pavlov IP (1941) Lectures on conditioned reflexes, vol 2. Lawrence Wishart, London
Pavlov IP (1955) Selected works. Foreign Languages Publishing House, Moscow
Phillips L, Zigler E (1961) Social competence: the action-thought parameter and vicariousness in normal and pathological behaviours. J Abnorm Soc Psychol 63: 137–146
Pilowsky I, Levine S, Boulton DM (1969) The classification of depression by numerical taxonomy. Br J Psychiatry 115: 937–945
Pinel P (1801) A treatise on insanity. Facsimile of the London 1806 edition. Hafner, New York 1962
Plaut A (1960) A concept of mental health. Br J Med Psychol 33: 275–278
Pollin W (1976) Genetic and environmental determinants of neurosis. In: Kaplan AR (ed) Human behaviour genetics. Thomas, Springfield, Ill.
Popper KR (1963) Conjectures and refutations. Routledge & Kegan Paul, London
Rabkin R (1964) Conversion hysteria as social maladaptation. Psychiatry 27: 349–363
Rachman S (1965) Aversion therapy: chemical or electrical? Behav Res & Ther 2: 289–299
Rachman S (1966) Studies in desensitisation: II. flooding. Behav Res Ther 4: 1–6
Rachman S (1972) Clinical applications of observational learning, imitation and modeling. Behav Ther 3: 379–397
Rachman S (1974) The meanings of fear. Penguin, Middlesex
Rachman S (1976) Obsessional-compulsive checking. Behav Res Ther 14: 269–277
Rachman S (1977) The conditioning theory of fear-acquisition: a critical examination. Behav Res Ther 15: 375–387
Rachman S, Hodgson RJ (1968) Experimentally-induced 'sexual fetishism': replication and development. Psychol Rec 18: 25–27
Rachman S, Hodgson R (1974) I. Synchrony and desynchrony in fear and avoidance. Behav Res Ther 12: 311–318
Rachman S, Hodgson R, Marks I (1971) Treatment of chronic obsessive-compulsive neuroses. Behav Res Ther 9: 237–247
Rachman S, Teasdale J (1969) Aversion therapy and behaviour disorders: an analysis. Routledge & Kegan Paul, London
Rachman S, Seligman MEP (1976) Unprepared phobias: "be prepared". Behav Res & Ther 14: 333–338
Ramsay RW (1975) Research on anxiety and phobic reactions. In: Spielberger CD, Sarason IG (eds) Stress and anxiety, vol 1. Hemisphere, Wiley, New York

Rescorla RA (1969) Establishment of a positive reinforcer through contrast with shock. J Comp Physiol Psychol 67: 260–263

Rogers CR (1965) Some thoughts regarding the current philosophy of the behavioural sciences. J Humanistic Psychol 5: 182–194

Rosen A (1962) Development of the MMPI scales based on a reference group of psychiatric patients. Psychol Monogr 76: 1–25

Rosenhan D (1973) On being sane in insane places. Science 179: 250–258

Roth M (1963) Neurosis, psychosis and the concept of disease in psychiatry. Acta Psychiatr Scand 39: 128–145

Rush AJ, Beck AT, Kovacs M, Hollon S (1977) Comparative efficacy of cognitive therapy and pharmacotherapy in the treatment of depressed outpatients. Cog Ther Res 1: 17–37

Rust J (1974) Genetic factors in psychophysiology. Unpublished PhD thesis, University of London, London

Rutter M, Korn S, Birch HG (1963) Genetic and environmental factors in the development of 'primary reaction patterns'. Br J Soc Clin Psychol 2: 161–173

Ryle A (1967) Neurosis in the ordinary family. Lippincott, Philadelphia

Sandifer MG (1977) The education of the psychiatrist as a physician. Am J Psychiatry 134: 50–53

Sandifer MG, Hordern A, Timbury GC, Green LM (1969) Similarities and differences in patient evaluation by US and UK psychiatrists. Am J Psychiatry 126: 206–212

Sanford N (1965) Will psychologists study human problems? Am Psychol 20: 192–207

Sarbin TR (1964) Anxiety: reification of a metaphor. Arch Gen Psychiatry 10: 630–638

Sartory G, Rachman S, Grey S (1977) An investigation of the relation between reported fear and heart rate. Behav Res Ther 15: 435–438

Sartory G, Lader M (1980) Psychophysiology and drugs in anxiety and phobias. In: Christie M, Mellett P (eds) Psychosomatic approaches in Medicine, vol 1. Behavioural approaches. Wiley, London

Saslow G, Peters AD (1956) A follow-up study of 'untreated' patients with various behaviour disorders. Psychiatr Quart 30: 283–302

Schachter S, Singer JE (1962) Cognitive, social and physiological determinants of emotional state. Psychol Rev 69: 379–399

Schachter S, Wheeler L (1962) Epinephrine, chlorpromazine and amusement. J Abnorm Soc Psychol 65: 121–128

Scheff TJ (1966) Being mentally ill. Weidenfeld & Nicolson, London

Scheier IH (1972) Anxiety at a distance. In: Dreger RM (ed) Multivariate personality research. Claitors, Baton Rouge

Schmidt HO, Fonda CP (1956) The reliability of psychiatric diagnosis: a new look. J Abnorm Soc Psychol 52: 262–267

Schoeneman (1977) The role of mental illness in the witch hunts of the seventeenth centuries: an assessment. J Hist Behav Sci 13: 337–351

Schofield M (1965) Sociological aspects of homosexuality. Longman, London

Sechenov IM (1863) Reflexes of the brain. Reprinted in Selected Works. Bookmiga, Moscow 1935

Sederer L (1977) Moral therapy and the problem of morale. Am J Psychiatry 134: 267–272

Seligman MEP (1970) On the generality of the laws of learning. Psychol Rev 77: 406–418

Seligman MEP (1971) Phobias and preparedness. Behav Ther 2: 307–320

Seligman MEP (1975) Helplessness: on depression, development and death. Freeman, San Francisco

Seligman MEP, Johnston JC (1973) A cognitive theory of avoidance learning. In: Guigan F, Lumsden D (eds) Contemporary approaches to conditioning and learning. Winston, Washington

Seligman MEP, Klein DC, Miller WR (1976) Depression. In: Leitenberg H (ed) Handbook of behaviour modification and behaviour therapy. Prentice Hall, New Jersey

Seligman MEP, Maier SF (1967) Failure to escape traumatic shock. J Exp Psychol 74: 1–9

Seligman MEP, Meyer B (1970) Chronic fear and ulcers in rats as a function of the unpredictability of safety. J Comp Physiol Psychol 73: 202–207

Selye H (1950) The physiology and pathology of exposure to stress. Acta Inc, Montreal

Selye H (1957) The stress of life. Longman, London

Shagass C, Jones AL (1958) A neurophysiological test for psychiatric diagnosis. Am J Psychiatry 114: 1002–1009

Shakow D (1965) The role of classification in the development of the science of psychopathology with particular reference to research. In: Katz MM, Cole JO, Barton WE (eds) The role and methodology of classification in psychiatry and psychopathology. US Government Printing Office, Washington, DC

Shaw BF (1977) Comparison of cognitive therapy and behaviour therapy in the treatment of depression. J Consult Clin Psychol 45: 543–551

Sheflen AE (1958) Analysis of thought model which persists in psychiatry. Psychosom Med 20: 235–241

Shepherd M (1973) The prevalence and distribution of psychiatric illness in general practice. J R Coll Gen Pract 23: 16–19

Shepherd M, Cooper B, Brown AC, Kalton G (1966) Psychiatric illness in general practice. Oxford University Press, London

Sherif M (1936) The psychology of social norms. Harper, New York

Shey HH (1971) Iatrogenic anxiety. Psychiatr Quart 45: 343–356

Shields J (1962) Monzygotic twins. Oxford University Press, London

Sidman M (1964) Anxiety. Proc Am Phil Soc 108: 478–481

Siegelman M (1978) Psychological adjustment of homosexual and heterosexual men: a cross-national replication. Arch Sex Behav 7: 1–11

Silver RJ, Sines LK (1961) MMPI characteristics of a state hospital population. J Clin Psychol 17: 142–146

Simon B (1972) Models of mind and mental illness in Ancient Greece: II. the Platonic model. J Hist Behav Sci 8: 389–404

Simon B (1973) Models of mind and mental illness in Ancient Greece: II. the Platonic model. J Hist Behav Sci 9: 3–17

Simon B, Weiner H (1966) Models of mind and mental illness in Ancient Greece: I. the Homeric model of mind. J Hist Behav Sci 2: 303–314

Slater E (1965) Diagnosis of 'hysteria'. Br Med J 1: 1395–1399

Slater E, Roth M (1969) Clinical psychiatry. Bailliere & Tindall Cassell, London

Slater E, Shields J (1969) Genetical aspects of anxiety. In: Lader MH (ed) Studies of anxiety. Headley, London

Solomon RL, Wynne LC (1953) Traumatic avoidance learning: acquisition in normal dogs. Psychol Monogr 67/354

Solomon RL, Wynne LC (1954) Traumatic avoidance learning: anxiety conservation and partial irreversibility. Psychol Rev 61: 353–385

Solomon RL, Turner LH, Lessac MS (1968) Some effects of delay of punishment on resistance to punishment in dogs. J Pers Soc Psychol 8: 233–238

Spence KW (1964) Anxiety (drive) level and performance in eyelid conditioning. Psychol Bull 61: 129–139

Spielberger CD, Gorsuch RL, Lushener RE (1968) The state-trait anxiety inventory. Florida State University, Florida

Stein M, Ottenberg P (1958) Role of odours in asthma. Psychosom Med 20: 60–65

Storms MD, McCaul KD (1976) Attributional processes and emotional exacerbation of dysfunctional behaviour. In: Harver JH, Ickes WJ, Kidd RF (eds) New directions in attribution research. Wiley, New York

Storms MD, Nisbett RE (1970) Insomnia and the attribution process. J Pers Soc Psychol 16: 319–328

Strauss JS (1975) A comprehensive approach to psychiatric diagnosis. Am J Psychiatry 132: 1193–1196

Stuart RB (1970) Trick or treatment: how and when psychotherapy fails. Research Press, Champaign, Ill.

Szasz TS (1960) The myth of mental illness. Am Psychol 15: 113–118

Szasz TS (1961) The myth of mental illness. Hoeber & Harper, New York

Taylor F Kraupl (1966) Psychopathology. Its causes and symptoms. Butterworths, London

Taylor JA (1953) A personality scale of manifest anxiety. J Abnorm Soc Psychol 48: 285–290

Teasdale J (1974) Learning models of obsessional-compulsive disorder. In: Beech HR (ed) Obsessional states. Methuen, London

Thomas A, Chess S, Birch HG (1968) Temperament and behaviour disorders in children. New York University Press, New York

Thompson C (1950) Psychoanalysis: evolution and development. Nelson, New York

Thomson R (1968) The pelican history of psychology. Penguin, Middlesex

Thorndike EL (1903) Educational psychology. Lemcke & Buechner, New York

Thorndike EL (1911) Animal intelligence. Macmillian, New York

Thorndike EL (1932) The fundamentals of learning. Teachers College, New York

Tolman EC (1948) Cognitive maps in rats and men. Psychol Rev 55: 189–208

Tredgold RF (1941) Depressive states in the soldier: their symptoms, causation and prognosis. Br Med J 2: 109–112

Trouton DS, Maxwell AE (1956) The relationship between neurosis and psychosis. J Ment Sci 102: 1–21

Trower PE, Yardley KM, Bryant BM, Shaw PH (1978) The treatment of social failure: a comparison of anxiety reduction and skills acquisition procedures on two social problems. Behav Mod 2, 41–60

Truax CB (1966) Reinforcement and non-reinforcement in Rogerian psychotherapy. J Abnorm Psychol 71: 1–9

Tuke S (1813) Description of The Retreat. Reprinted 1964. Dawson, London

Ullman LP, Krasner L (1967) The psychological model. In: Millon T (ed) Theories of psychopathology. Saunders, Philadelphia

Ullman LP, Krasner L (1969) A psychological approach to abnormal behaviour. Prentice-Hall, New Jersey

Valins S (1966) Cognitive effects of false heart-rate feedback. J Pers Soc Psychol 4: 400–408

Valins S, Nisbett RE, Jones EE, Kanouse DE, Kelley HE, Weiner B (1971) Attribution processes in the development and treatment of emotional disorders. In: Jones et al. (eds) Attribution. General Learning Press, New Jersey

Vandenberg SG, Clark PJ, Samuels I (1965) Psychophysiological reactions of twins: heritability factors in galvanic skin resistance, heartbeat, and breathing rates. Eugen Quart 12: 7–10

Wallace HER, Whyte MBH (1959) Natural history of the psychoneuroses. Br Med J 1: 144–148

Ward CH, Beck AT, Mendelson M, Mock JE, Erbaugh JK (1962) The psychiatric nomenclature: reasons for diagnostic disagreement. Arch Gen Psychiatry 7: 198–205

Warner EC (1952) Savill's system of clinical medicine. Arnold, London

Watson JB (1930) Behaviourism. Kegan Paul & Trench Trubner, London

Watson JB, Rayner R (1920) Conditioned emotional reactions. J Exp Psychol 3: 1–14

Weiss E (1942) Anxiety and the heart. Clinics 1: 916–931

Weiss JM (1968) Effects of coping responses on stress. J Comp Physiol Psychol 65: 251–260

Weiss JM, Glazer HI, Pohorecky LA (1976) Coping behaviour and neurochemical changes. In: Serban G, Kling A (eds) Animal models in human psychobiology. Plenum, New York

Wexler M (1971) Schizophrenia: conflict and deficiency. Psychoanal Q 40: 83–99

Wilde GJS (1964) Inheritance of personality traits. Acta Psychol 22: 37–51

Williams HV, Lipman RS, Rickels K, Covi L, Uhlenhuth EH, Mattsson NB (1968) Replication of symptom distress factors in anxious neurotic outpatients. Multivar Behav Res 3: 199–211

Willis MH, Blaney PH (1978) Three tests of the learned helplessness model of depression. J Abnorm Psychol 87: 131–136

Wing JK (1973) Social and familial factors in the causation and treatment of schizophrenia. In: Iverson LL, Rose SPR (eds) Biochemistry and mental illness. Biochemical Society, London

Wing JK, Cooper JE, Sartorius N (1974) The measurement and classification of psychiatric symptoms. Cambridge University Press, London

Wing L (1964) Physiological effects of performing a difficult task in patients with anxiety states. J Psychosom Res 7: 283–294

Wolpe J (1952) Experimental neurosis as learned behaviour. Br J Psychol 43: 243–261

Wolpe J (1958) Psychotherapy by reciprocal inhibition. Stanford University Press, Stanford, Ca.

Wolpe J (1960) Reciprocal inhibition as the main basis of psychotherapeutic effects. In: Eysenck HJ (ed) Behaviour therapy and the neuroses. Pergamon, London

Wolpe J (1967a) Etiology of human neuroses. In: Millon T (ed) Theories of psychopathology. Saunders, London

Wolpe J (1967b) Parallels between animal and human neuroses. In: Zubin J, Hunt HF (eds) Comparative psychopathology. Grune & Stratton, New York

Wolpe J (1968) Learning theories. In: Howells JG (ed) Modern perspectives in world psychiatry. Oliver Boyd, London

Wolpe J (1970) The experimental foundations of some new psychotherapeutic methods. In: Gantt WH, Pickerhain L, Zwingmann C (eds) Pavlovian approach to psychopathology. Pergamon, London

Wolpe J (1978) Cognition and causation in human behaviour and its therapy. Am Psychol 33: 437–446

Wolpe J, Brady JP, Serber M, Agras WS, Liberman RP (1973) The current status of systematic desensitisation. Am J Psychiatry 130: 961–965

Wolpe J, Rachman S (1960) Psychoanalytic 'evidence': a critique based on Freud's case of Little Hans. J Nerv Ment Dis 130: 135–148

Wortman CB, Dintzer L (1978) Is an attributional analysis of the learned helplessness phenomenon viable? J Abnorm Psychol 87: 75–90

Wortman CB, Panciera L, Shusterman L, Hibscher J (1976) Attributions of causality and reactions to uncontrollable outcomes. J Exp Soc Psychol 12: 301–316

Wyss D (1966) Depth psychology: a critical history. Allen & Unwin, London

Yarrow M, Schwartz C, Murphy H, Deasy L (1955) The psychological meaning of mental illness in the family. J Soc Iss 11: 12–24

Yates AJ (1958) Symptoms and symptom substitution. Psychol Rev 65: 371–374

Yates AJ (1975) Theory and practice in behaviour therapy. Wiley, New York

Zajonj RB (1965) Social facilitation. Science 149: 269–274

Zilboorg G, Henry GW (1941) A History of medical psychology. Norton, New York

Zubin J (1967) Classification of the behaviour disorders. Annu Rev Psychol 18: 373–406

11. Author Index

12. Subject Index

W. H. Gaddes
Learning Disabilities and Brain Function
A Neuropsychological Approach
With a Foreword by W. M. Cruickshank
1980. 45 figures, 4 tables. XVI, 403 pages
ISBN 3-540-90486-7

Contents: Neurology and Behavior: Some Professional Problems. – Prevalence Estimates and Etiology of Learning Disabilities. – The Nervous System and Learning. – The Use of Neuropsychological Knowledge in Understanding Learning. Disorders. – Perceptual Disorders. – Sensory and Motor Pathways and Learning. – Cerebral Dominance, Handedness, and Laterality. – Languange Development, Aphasia, and Dyslexia. – The Neuropsychological Basis of Problems in Writing, Spelling, and Arithmetic. – Remediation, Therapy, and the Learning-Disabled Child. – Postscript. – Appendices. – Glossary. – References. – Indexes.

Neural Mechanisms in Behavior
A Texas Symposium
Editor: D. McFadden
With contributions by H. B. Barlow, R. M. Boynton, E. V. Evarts, E. R. Kandel, F. Ratliff, J. E. Rose, R. F. Thompson
1980. 151 figures, 1 table. XI, 308 pages
ISBN 3-540-90468-9

Contents: Neural Correlates of Some Psychoacoustic Experiences. – Design for an Eye. – Form and Function: Linear and Nonlinear Analyses of Neural Networks in the Visual System. – Cortical Function: A Tentative Theory and Preliminary Tests. – The Search for the Engram, II. – Brain Mechanisms in Voluntary Movement. – Cellular Insight into the Multivariant Nature of Arousal. – General Discussion. – Index.

D. W. Pfaff
Estrogens and Brain Function
Neural Analysis of a Hormone-Controlled Mammalian Reproductive Behavior
1980. 109 figures, 1 color plate, 20 tables. X, 281 pages
ISBN 3-540-90487-5

Contents: Introduction. – Triggering the Behavior: Sensory and Ascending Pathways: Stimulus. Primary Sensory Neurons. Spinal Interneurons. Ascending Neural Pathways. – Facilitating the Behavior: Sex Hormones in the Brain: Steroid Sex Hormone Binding by Cells in the the Vertebrate Brain. Hypothalamic Mechanisms. Hypothalamic Outflow. Midbrain Module. – Executive Control over the Behavior: Descending and Motor Pathways: Brainstem to Spinal Cord. Motoneurons and Response Execution. – Building on this Paradigm: Logical and Heuristic Developments. – Summary. Epiloque. – References.

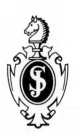

Springer-Verlag
Berlin
Heidelberg
New York

J. C. Eccles

The Human Psyche

The GIFFORD Lectures
University of Edinburgh 1978–1979

1980. 76 figures, 2 tables. XV, 279 pages
ISBN 3-540-09954-9

H. J. Eysenck

The Structure and Measurement of Intelligence

With Contributions by D. W. Fulker

1979. 69 figures, 38 tables. V, 253 pages
ISBN 3-540-09028-2

W. W. Henton, I. H. Iversen

Classical Conditioning and Operant Conditioning

A Response Pattern Analysis

1978. 106 figures, 16 tables. XVII, 355 pages
ISBN 3-540-09326-7

J. P. Henry, P. M. Stephens

Stress, Health, and the Social Environment

A Sociobiologic Approach to Medicine

1977. 171 figures. XII, 282 pages
(Topics in Environmental Physiology and Medicine)
ISBN 3-540-90293-7

K. R. Popper, J. C. Eccles

The Self and Its Brain

1977. 66 figures. XVI, 597 pages
ISBN 3-540-08307-3
Distribution rights for Great Britain: Global Book
Resources of Henley-on-Thames

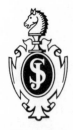

Springer-Verlag
Berlin
Heidelberg
New York

E. Székely

Functional Laws of Psychodynamics

1979. 63 figures, 10 tables. VIII, 353 pages
ISBN 3-540-90371-2